Ketogenic Diet for Beginners Guide

Congratulations on taking charge of your health and wellness by choosing to start a ketogenic (keto) diet. While you may know that a ketogenic diet is a low-carbohydrate way of eating, there is much to learn about how it works and what you can do to successfully follow it. Enjoy reading!!

The Keto diet involves going long spells on extremely low (no higher than 30g per day) to almost zero g per day of carbs and increasing your fats to a really high level (to the point where they may make up as much as 65% of your daily macronutrients intake.) The idea behind this is to get your body into a state of ketosis. In this state of ketosis the body is supposed to be more inclined to use fat for energy- and research says it does just this. Depleting your carbohydrate/glycogen liver stores and then moving onto fat for fuel means you should end up being shredded.

You then follow this basic platform from say Monday until Sat 12pm (afternoon) (or Sat 7pm, depending on whose version you read). Then from this time until 12 midnight Sunday night (so up to 36 hours later) do your massive carb up...

(Some say, and this will also be dictated by your body type, that you can go nuts in the carb up and eat anything you want and then there are those that more wisely- in my view- prescribe still sticking to the clean carbs even during your carb up.)

So calculating your numbers is as simple as the following...

Calculate your required maintenance level of daily calories...

(if you are looking to drop quickly use 13- I would not advise this, if you want a more level drop in body fat use 15 and if you are going to actually attempt to maintain or possibly put on some lean muscle mass then use 17)

Body weight in pounds x 15= a

Protein for the day 1g per body weight in pounds= b

Bx4=c (c= number of calories allotted to your daily protein allowance).

a-c= d (d= amount of calories to be allotted to fat intake).

D/9= g per day of fat to be consumed.

The end calculation should leave you with a very high number for your fat intake.

Now for those of you wondering about energy levels... Especially for training because there are no carbs, with there being such a high amount of fat in the diet you feel quite full and the fat is a very good fuel source for your body. (One adaptation that I have made is to actually have a nice fish fillet about an hour before I train and I find it gives me enough energy to get through my workout.) (I am aware of the arguments made to not have fats 2-3 hrs otherwise of training. While I won't have fats 2-3 hrs after training as I want □uick absorption and blood flow then, I see no issue with slowing everything down before training so my body has access to a slow digesting energy source).

There are some that say to have a 30g carb intake immediately after training- just enough to fill liver glycogen levels. And then there are those that say having even as much as that may push you out of ketosis- the state you are trying to maintain. As I have done the post-workout shake for the last 8+ years of my training I have decided to try the "no post-workout" route! I figure I may as well try!

During my carb up period- for the sake of those who would like to know of you can get in shape and sill eat the things you want (in moderation)- for the first six weeks I will be relaxed about what I eat in this period but then the following 6 weeks I will only eat clean carbs.

I also like to make sure that the first workout of the week- as in a Monday morning workout- is a nice long full hour of work so I start cutting into the liver glycogen already.

I also make sure to have one last really grueling workout on Saturday before my carb up.

USES AND BENEFITS OF THE KETOGENIC DIET

When using a ketogenic diet, your body becomes more of a fat-burner than a carbohydrate-dependent machine. Several researches have linked the consumption of increased amounts of carbohydrates to development of several disorders such as diabetes and insulin resistance.

By nature, carbohydrates are easily absorbable and therefore can be also be easily stored by the body. Digestion of carbohydrates starts right from the moment you put them into your mouth.

As soon as you begin chewing them, amylase (the enzymes that digest carbohydrate) in your saliva is already at work acting on the carbohydrate-containing food.

In the stomach, carbohydrates are further broken down. When they get into the small intestines, they are then absorbed into the bloodstream. On getting to the bloodstream, carbohydrates generally increase the blood sugar level.

This increase in blood sugar level stimulates the immediate release of insulin into the bloodstream. The higher the increase in blood sugar levels, the more the amount of insulin that is release.

Insulin is a hormone that causes excess sugar in the bloodstream to be removed in order to lower the blood sugar level. Insulin takes the sugar and carbohydrate that you eat and stores them either as glycogen in muscle tissues or as fat in adipose tissue for future use as energy.

However, the body can develop what is known as insulin resistance when it is continuously exposed to such high amounts of glucose in the bloodstream. This scenario can easily cause obesity as the body tends to □uickly store any excess amount of glucose. Health conditions such as diabetes and cardiovascular disease can also result from this condition.

Keto diets are low in carbohydrate and high in fat and have been associated with reducing and improving several health conditions.

One of the foremost things a ketogenic diet does is to stabilize your insulin levels and also restore leptin signalling. Reduced amounts of insulin in the bloodstream allow you to feel fuller for a longer period of time and also to have fewer cravings.

Medical Benefits of Ketogenic Diets

The application and implementation of the ketogenic diet has expanded considerably. Keto diets are often indicated as part of the treatment plan in a number of medical conditions.

Epilepsy

This is basically the main reason for the development of the ketogenic diet. For some reason, the rate of epileptic seizures reduces when patients are placed on a keto diet.

Pediatric epileptic cases are the most responsive to the keto diet. There are children who have experience seizure elimination after a few years of using a keto diet.

Children with epilepsy are generally expected to fast for a few days before starting the ketogenic diet as part of their treatment.

Cancer

Research suggests that the therapeutic efficacy of the ketogenic diets against tumor growth can be enhanced when combined with certain drugs and procedures under a "press-pulse" paradigm.

It is also promising to note that ketogenic diets drive the cancer cell into remission. This means that keto diets "starves cancer" to reduce the symptoms.

Alzheimer Disease

There are several indications that the memory functions of patients with Alzheimer's disease improve after making use of a ketogenic diet.

Ketones are a great source of alternative energy for the brain especially when it has become resistant to insulin. Ketones also provide substrates (cholesterol) that help to repair damaged neurons and membranes. These all help to improve memory and cognition in Alzheimer patients.

Diabetes

It is generally agreed that carbohydrates are the main culprit in diabetes. Therefore, by reducing the amount of ingested carbohydrate by using a ketogenic diet, there are increased chances for improved blood sugar control.

Also, combining a keto diet with other diabetes treatment plans can significantly improve their overall effectiveness.

Gluten Allergy

Many individuals with gluten allergy are undiagnosed with this condition. However, following a ketogenic diet showed improvement in related symptoms like digestive discomforts and bloating.

Most carbohydrate-rich foods are high in gluten. Thus, by using a keto diet, a lot of the gluten consumption is reduced to a minimum due to the elimination of a large variety of carbohydrates.

Weight Loss

This is arguably the most common "intentional" use of the ketogenic diet today. It has found a niche for itself in the mainstream dieting trend. Keto diets have become part of many dieting regimen due to its well acknowledged side effect of aiding weight loss.

Though initially maligned by many, the growing number of favorable weight loss results has helped the ketogenic to better embraced as a major weight loss program.

Besides the above medical benefits, ketogenic diets also provide some general health benefits which include the following.

Improved Insulin Sensitivity

This is obviously the first aim of a ketogenic diet. It helps to stabilize your insulin levels thereby improving fat burning.

Muscle Preservation

Since protein is oxidized, it helps to preserve lean muscle. Losing lean muscle mass causes an individual's metabolism to slow down as muscles are generally very metabolic. Using a keto diet actually helps to preserve your muscles while your body burns fat.

Controlled pH and respiratory function

A ketoc diet helps to decrease lactate thereby improving both pH and respiratory function. A state of ketosis therefore helps to keep your blood pH at a healthy level.

Improved Immune System

Using a ketogenic diet helps to fight off aging antioxidants while also reducing inflammation of the gut thereby making your immune system stronger.

Reduced Cholesterol Levels

Consuming fewer carbohydrates while you are on the keto diet will help to reduce blood cholesterol levels. This is due to the increased state of lipolysis. This leads to a reduction in LDL cholesterol levels and an increase in HDL cholesterol levels.

Reduced Appetite and Cravings

Adopting a ketogenic diet helps you to reduce both your appetite and cravings for calorie rich foods. As you begin eating healthy, satisfying, and beneficial high-fat foods, your hunger feelings will naturally start decreasing.

THE DIFFERENCES BETWEEN KETO AND PALEO DIETS

Obesity rivals smoking as the number one cause of preventable death. One reason is the dramatic rise in the diabetes risk often accompanying weight gain. So, are you interested in starting up a new diet plan, one aimed to not only help you lose weight but to control your blood sugar better? Chances are you are searching for the best options available. Two you may come across as they are trendy in today's times are the ketogenic diet and the paleo diet. Many people actually get confused between these as they do tend to be similar so it can be hard to differentiate between them.

Let us compare so you can see which one is right for you...

Carb Sources. First, let's talk carb sources as this is where the two diets vastly differ...

with the paleo diet plan, your carb sources are going to be any fresh fruit, along with sweet potatoes. Together, you can quickly achieve 100 grams or more of carbohydrates between these two foods.

the keto diet, on the other hand, your only carb source is leafy greens, and even those are restricted.

So one of the most significant differences between the ketogenic diet and the paleo diet plan is the ketogenic diet is deficient in carbohydrates while the paleo is not. You can make the paleo diet very low carb if you want, but it is not by default. There is more flexibility in food choices.

Calorie Counting. Next, we come to calorie counting. This is also a place where the two diets differ considerably.

With the keto diet, you will be calorie and macro counting Quite heavily. You need to hit specific targets...

30% total protein intake,

5% carbohydrate intake and

65% dietary fat intake.

If you do not reach these targets, you are not going to move into the "state of ketosis," which is the entire point of this diet plan.

With the paleo diet, there are no strict rules around this. While you can count calories if you want, you do not have to. Obviously, your fat loss results will likely be better if you do monitor calories to some degree since calories do dictate whether you gain or lose body fat, but it is not essential.

Exercise Fuel Availability. Which brings us to our next point - exercise fuel availability. To be able to exercise with intensity, you need carbohydrates in your diet plan. You cannot get fuel availability if you are not eating carbohydrate-rich foods - that means the keto diet is not going to support intense exercise sessions. For this reason, the keto diet will not be optimal for most people. Exercise is an integral part of staying healthy, so it is strongly recommended you exercise and do not follow a diet that limits exercise.

Of course, you can do the targeted ketogenic diet or the cyclic ketogenic diet, both of which have you including carbohydrates in the diet at some point...

the targeted ketogenic diet has you eating carbohydrates just before starting your workout session while

the cyclic ketogenic diet calls for you to eat a larger dose of carbs over the weekend, which are designed to sustain you through the rest of the week.

If you follow either of these, you can choose any carbohydrates you wish; it does not necessarily have to be just sweet potatoes or fruit.

There you have some critical differences between these two approaches...

the ketogenic diet is one focusing more on tracking macros and is intended to assist with fat loss while

the paleo diet focuses more on good food choices and health and hopes weight loss comes as a result.

Although managing Type 2 diabetes can be very challenging, it is not a condition you must just live with. Make simple changes to your daily routine - include exercise to help lower both your blood sugar levels and your weight.

FOR EXERCISING WHEN ON A KETOGENIC DIET

A lot of things happen when you are exercising. Some of these are good for your health and others are not so good - like when you exercise excessively.

Exercise is a stressor. While it can be a good stressor, it can however cause your adrenals to go into overdrive. This situation increases your insulin levels and therefore reduces your ability to lose weight.

When exercising, your insulin levels goes up while your hunger reduces. However, this often results in a significant reduction in blood sugar levels which results to you becoming hungrier.

It is important to note that even a moderate increase in insulin levels causes a significant lowering of fat loss or lipolysis.

One problem we have when we want to lose weight is that we focus so much on the numbers showing on the scale. We almost unconsciously forget about the most important thing which is losing body fat.

We have more than 80 percent of our body fat stored in fat cells. To be able to get rid of these stored fat, one would need to burn it for energy production.

However, before your body can start burning your stored fats for energy, your need to be in a negative fat balance. This is condition in which you are burning more fat off than you are actually taking in through your diet.

If your body has become used to burning fat for energy, it can now use both body fat and dietary fat for energy. This is one of the key powers of using a ketogenic diet for losing weight.

If you do not increase your dietary fat intake but increase the amount of energy your body needs through increasing your exercise intensity, your body will get almost all of that energy from burning body fat.

However, if your body is fueled with carbs, you will mostly be burning glucose for energy. This makes it a lot difficult for your body to burn and lose body fat.

It is however important to understand that while exercise can help you lose weight, it is more important to get the diet right first.

When you get the diet right, such a by using a well-designed ketogenic diet, your body will start tapping into its fat deposits for generating its energy. This is what effectively enables you to start burning and losing body fat.

Once your body gets used to the ketogenic diet, you will start feeling more energetic. At such a point, you will be better positioned to adjust your menus in order to start building strength and muscles.

When you get to this point during the "standard ketogenic" diet, you can then alter the diet to either a "targeted" or a "cyclical" ketogenic diet. These versions of the ketogenic diet allow more carbohydrate consumption to enable you engage in more exercises for longer.

Targeted Ketogenic Diet

The Targeted Ketogenic Diet allows you to ingest more carbs around your exercise period. This form of the diet allows you to engage in high-intensity exercise while still remaining in ketosis.

The carb intake within this window provides your muscles with the necessary glucose to effectively engage in your workouts. The extra glucose should normally be used up during this window of about 30 minutes and should not affect your overall metabolism.

The Targeted Ketogenic Diet is designed for beginners or intermittent exercisers. The TKD allows a slight increase in your carb consumption. However, it does not kick you out ketosis and causes no shock to your system.

Cyclical Ketogenic Diet

The Cyclical Ketogenic Diet is more appropriate for advanced athletes and bodybuilders. It is generally used for maximum muscle building results.

There is however a strong tendency for other individuals to end up adding some body fat. This is because it is easy to overeat while using the Cyclical Ketogenic Diet (CKD).

In this version of the ketogenic diet, the individual follows the standard ketogenic diet for 5 or 6 days. He or she is then allowed to eat increased amounts of carbohydrate for 1 or 2 days.

As a caution, it can take a beginner close to 3 weeks to fully get back into ketosis if he or she attempts the CKD. It requires real commitment and advanced exercise levels to successfully carry out a CKD.

The aim of the Cyclical Ketogenic Diet is to temporarily switch out of ketosis. This window gives the body the opportunity to refill the amount of glycogen in the muscles to enable it undertake the next cycle of intense workouts.

Therefore, there must be a complete depletion of the resultant glycogen build up during the subsequent workouts in order to get back into ketosis. The intensity of your planned workout will consequently determine the amount of increased carbohydrate intake.

Cardio Exercises

When you exercise at an intense rate, a lot of amazing things happen to your body.

When you engage in cardiovascular exercises, they help to improve the efficiency of your heart and lungs. This also helps to increase the rate at which your body burns energy and over time this will lead to weight loss.

Engaging in cardio exercise causes many metabolic changes that positively affect fat metabolism.

Cardiovascular exercises helps to increase oxygen delivery through improved blood flow. This way, body cells are able to more effectively oxidize and burn fat.

This also has the effect of increasing the number of oxidative enzymes. Consequently, the speed at which fatty acids are transported to the mitochondria to be burned for energy is greatly increased.

During cardio exercises, the sensitivity of muscles and fat cells to epinephrine is greatly increased. This increases the amount of triglycerides that are released into the blood and muscles to be burned for energy.

Strength Training

Strength training helps to improve your moods while also helping to build healthy bones. It also helps you to develop an overall strong and healthy body.

Using a well-designed ketogenic will help you preserve your muscles even when carrying our strength training. Muscles are built with protein and not fat or carbs. Also, given the fact that protein oxidation is less in a ketogenic diet, engaging in strength training should not be a problem.

You need to challenge your body with heavy weights to really see results and get a stronger body.

Interval Training

Interval training is simply alternating intervals of high-intensity and low-intensity workouts. It is simply for you to: go fast, go slow, and repeat.

While sounding so simple, interval training is one the most powerful ways to burn body fat quickly. Apart from burning fat while carrying out interval training, the "afterburn effect" stimulates your metabolism for a longer period of time.

Circuit Training: Cardio + Strength

Circuit training is basically the combining of cardiovascular exercises with strength training exercises. This combination helps to provide all-over fitness benefits.

This form of exercising combines cardio exercises such a jogging and a resistance workout without allowing a resting period between them. The lack of rest in-between both exercises make circuit training as effective as a cardio-based high-intensity interval training workout.

Yoga

The exercise benefits of yoga really come from its ability to help the body reduce levels of stress hormones and also increase insulin sensitivity.

Yoga helps you to consciously connect with your body. This connection can translate into you being more mindful of how your body works and changing even your eating habits.

HERE ARE 10 FOODS YOU MUST HAVE IN YOUR KITCHEN

The ketogenic diet is a very successful weight-loss program. It utilizes high fat and low carbohydrate ingredients in order to burn fat instead of glucose. Many people are familiar with the Atkins diet, but the keto plan restricts carbs even more.

Because we are surrounded by fast food restaurants and processed meals, it can be a challenge to avoid carb-rich foods, but proper planning can help.

Plan menus and snacks at least a week ahead of time, so you aren't caught with only high carb meal choices. Research keto recipes online; there are Quite a few good ones to choose from. Immerse yourself in the keto lifestyle, find your favorite recipes, and stick with them.

There are a few items that are staples of a keto diet. Be sure to have these items on hand:

- **Eggs** - Used in omelets, Quiches (yes, heavy cream is legal on keto!), hard boiled as a snack, low carb pizza crust, and more; if you like eggs, you have a great chance of success on this diet

- **Bacon** - Do I need a reason? breakfast, salad garnish, burger topper, BLT's (no bread of course; try a BLT in a bowl, tossed in mayo)

- **Cream cheese** - Dozens of recipes, pizza crusts, main dishes, desserts

- **Shredded cheese** - Sprinkle over taco meat in a bowl, made into tortilla chips in the microwave, salad toppers, low-carb pizza and enchiladas

- **Lots of romaine and spinach** - Fill up on the green veggies; have plenty on hand for a ⬜uick salad when hunger pangs hit

- **EZ-Sweetz liquid sweetener** - Use a couple of drops in place of sugar; this artificial sweetener is the most natural and easiest to use that I've found

- **Cauliflower** - Fresh or frozen bags you can eat this low-carb veggie by itself, tossed in olive oil and baked, mashed in fake potatoes, chopped/shredded and used in place of rice under main dishes, in low-carb and keto pizza crusts, and much more

- **Frozen chicken tenders** - Have a large bag on hand; thaw quickly and grill, saute, mix with veggies and top with garlic sauce in a low carb flatbread, use in Chicken piccata, chicken alfredo, tacos, enchiladas, Indian Butter chicken, and more

- **Ground beef** - Make a big burger and top with all sorts of things from cheese, to sauteed mushrooms, to grilled onions... or crumble and cook with taco seasoning and use in provolone cheese taco shells; throw in a dish with lettuce, avocado, cheese, sour cream for a tortilla-less taco salad

- **Almonds (plain or flavored)** - these are a tasty and healthy snack; however, be sure to count them as you eat, because the carbs DO add up. Flavors include habanero, coconut, salt and vinegar and more.

The keto plan is a versatile and interesting way to lose weight, with lots of delicious food choices. Keep these 10 items stocked in your fridge, freezer, and larder, and you'll be ready to throw together some delicious keto meals and snacks at a moment's notice.

The ketogenic diet is a healthy option for anyone who wants to lose weight. Visit the Healthy Keto website, a valuable resource where keto dieters can access meal ideas and keto diet facts.

HOW TO EAT SUCCESFULLY AT RESTAURANTS

For those who eat low-carb or keto diets, there is almost always something you can eat in every fast food place or restaurant. Plan ahead. Before entering a restaurant, check out their menu and nutrition information online at home or using your smart phone. It's always good to know the safe options before being tempted by menu items you shouldn't have on a low-carb diet.

In order to make it easier to find a quick keto-friendly option, I've compiled a list of several restaurants and fast food places and those items that I've found to be the lowest carb (and most emotionally satisfying) choices. These are not all perfect options, but when you're stuck with no other choices due to time or location constraints, they'll do in a pinch.

It's a huge help that fast-food places are required to post nutritional content. It gets easier to follow the keto plan every day. The carb count I'm listing is approximate and is NET grams.

In general, there is usually some salad option anywhere you are. At Burger joints, just remove the bun, and many places offer lettuce wraps instead. Chicken shouldn't have breading.

As a side note, it helps to have a knife and fork handy in your car or purse. Big, juicy burgers in tiny pieces of lettuce end up on the table - or in your lap. Small, flimsy fastfood plasticware also makes for difficult eating. Pull out your own sturdy utensils and enjoy!

Now for the food choices... here are some pretty obvious general rules to follow:

Skip the bun or wrap

Skip the pasta, potato, or rice

Salads - no croutons. Stick with low sugar dressing options - Caesar, Blue Cheese, Ranch, Chipotle. Look at the name which may give you a clue, things like "honey" in the honey dijon or "sweet" in the dressing name - these are usually not a good choice. Check the ingredient for items that are higher in carb content.

Chicken - Choose grilled or sauteed. Stay away from any chicken that is breaded.

McDonald's - opt for any burger (zero g) or grilled chicken (2 g) without the bun and topped with cheese, mayo, mustard, onions, etc. No ketchup. Add a side salad (3g). The Caesar salad with grilled chicken or the bacon ranch salad with grilled chicken are 9g.

Burger King - same burger info as McDonald's: burger (zero g) without the bun and topped with cheese, mayo, mustard, onions, etc. No ketchup. The tendergrill chicken sandwich without the bun is 3g. BEWARE - you might think the veggie burger is low, but it is 19g of carbs, so that's about a full day of carbs on keto. Add a side salad (3g). The tendergrill chicken garden salad is 8g without dressing or croutons. The tendercrisp chicken salad is not an option. Do not attempt.

BONUS - dessert!?! - the fresh apple fries are not fried and are 5g net carbs WITHOUT caramel sauce.

Subway - Probably should skip Subway if you can. The buns and wraps are all high in carbs. I guess you could just have them throw the ingredients in a wrapper sans bun, but that doesn't sound appealing. I have no info on what the carb count would be for each bunless sub, but you can probably figure it out - chicken or pepperoni is fine, but is "sweet onion" chicken okay? No idea. Stick to the salads, but realize you'll only get iceberg lettuce (4g).

Carl's Junior and Hardees - This chain offers "lettuce wraps" - your burger wrapped in a large piece of lettuce for easy low carb eating. (As I've said, I tried it and don't love it. I like to carry my own fork instead.) Bunless options - Six dollar burger (7g), 1/2 thick-burger (5g), charbroiled chicken club sandwich (7g/10g at Hardees). Grilled chicken salad without croutons is 10g. Side salad is 3g.

Jimmy John's - The unwich - a sandwich wrapped in lettuce - fits the bill here. Meats are fine, just make sure the ingredients are not carb-rich.

Wendy's - Again, you can get your burger in a lettuce wrap or a box. Any burger with toppings. Mayo has corn syrup, and is 1g. The chicken grill fillet is 1 g. It can be ordered in the chicken club sandwich or the ultimate chicken grill sandwich. Best salads: chicken caesar (7g), blt chicken salad with grilled chicken. Side salads aer 6g or 2g for Caesar.

Pizza Hut and other pizza places - It is possible to get used to eating pizza with no crust. You need to eat twice as much, but if there's a party or dinner out that you can't avoid at a pizza place, just slide the cheesy toppings off and eat the big messy pile of cheese and toppings. A side salad is a nice addition. Otherwise, just opt for making pizza at home with a low-carb crust.

Mongolian Barbecue - YES! Load up your bowl with chicken, shrimp, onion slices, and mushrooms, then top with the Asian black bean sauce. I know beans have carbs, but this sauce label says 1 gram of carbs per ounce (each sauce is plainly labeled). Add a bit of garlic and wait for the griller to do his work. It goes without saying that you skip the appetizers, tortillas, and rice. Ask the wait staff not to bring them to the table.

Italian Restaurants - These take a little cunning, but they can be conqurerd! Ideas: how about chicken Marsala in an Italian place? Make sure it doesn't come with pasta. Substitute broccoli or some other keto-friendly side dish - or a big salad. Chicken piccata is also a possibility.

Mexican and Chinese restaurants are the most difficult, because any low carb option is not the reason to go to the restaurant in the first place. At a Mexican restaurant, I tend to get a large burrito with no beans and spread the soft tortilla out like a plate. Eat the inner ingredients and toss the tortilla.

If you MUST go to a Chinese buffet (I attended a funeral dinner at one), you can find options, but they probably aren't going to be your favorite General Tso's. How about the salad bar choices? eggs? the insides of eggrolls, and I even ate the insides only of crab rangoons. Unfortunately, these ideas leave □uite a pile of discarded shells and deep fried exterior pieces on your plate and makes it look like you really waste food.

Wings anywhere - Standard buffalo sauce is usually OK as well as garlic Parmesan

Convenience stores can be a good option, too! 7-11 has packs of hard boiled eggs, cheese slabs, slim jims, almonds, and pork rinds. Pork rinds come in a barbecue flavor and they're ZERO carbs.

Remember, whatever you choose, hold the bread, potatoes, rice, noodles, fries, and tortillas. And watch out for the possibility of corn starch, bread crumbs, and other fillers. With proper planning and a good attitude, you can find healthy keto and low-carb options when dining out, and stick to your successful keto diet plan.

The ketogenic diet is a healthy option for anyone who wants to lose weight. Visit the Healthy Keto website, a valuable resource where keto dieters can access meal ideas and keto diet facts.

The keto diet. What is the keto diet? In simple terms it's when you trick your body into using your own BODYFAT as it's main energy source instead of carbohydrates. The keto diet is very popular method of losing fat □uickly and efficiently.

The Science Behind It

To get your body into a ketogenic state you must eat a high fat diet and low protein with NO carbs or hardly any. The ratio should be around 80% fat and 20% protein. This will the guideline for the first 2 days. Once in a ketogenic state you will have to increase protein intake and lower fat, ratio will be around 65% fat, 30% protein and 5% carbs. Protein is increased to spare muscle tissue. When your body intakes carbohydrates it causes an insulin spike which means the pancreas releases insulin (helps store glycogen, amino acids and excess calories as fat) so common sense tells us that if we eliminate carbs then the insulin will not store excess calories as fat. Perfect.

Now your body has no carbs as a energy source your body must find a new source. Fat. This works out perfectly if you want to lose body fat. The body will break down the body fat and use it as energy instead of carbs. This state is called ketosis. This is the state you want your body to be in, makes perfect sense if you want to lose body fat while maintaining muscle.

Now to the diet part and how to plan it. You will need to intake AT LEAST a gram of protein per pounds of LEAN MASS. This will help in the recovery and repair of muscle tissue after workouts and such. Remember the ratio? 65% fat and 30% protein. Well if you weight 150 pounds of lean mass which means 150g of protein a day. X4 (amount of calories per gram of protein) that is 600 calories. The rest of your calories should come from fat. If your caloric maintenance is 3000 you must eat around 500 less which would mean that if you need 2500 calories a day, around 1900 calories must come from fats! You must eat fats to fuel your body which in return will also burn off body fat! That is the rule of this diet, you must eat fats! The advantage to eating dietary fats and the keto diet is that you will not feel hungry. Fat digestion is slow which works to your advantage and helps you feel 'full'.

You will be doing this monday - friday and then " carb-up " on the weekend. After your last workout on friday this is when the carb up starts. You must intake a liquid carbohydrate along with your whey shake post workout. This helps create an insulin spike and helps get the nutrients your body desperately needs for muscle repair and growth and refill glycogen stores. During this stage (carb up) eat what you want - pizzas, pasta, crisps, ice cream. Anything. This will be beneficial for you because it will refuel your body for the upcoming week as well as restoring your body's nutrient needs. Once sunday starts its back to the no carb high fat moderate protein diet. Keeping your body in ketosis and burning fat as energy is the perfect solution.

Another advantage to ketosis is once your get into the state of ketosis and burn off the fat you'r body will be depleted of carbs. Once you load up with carbs you will look as full as ever (with less bodyfat!) which is perfect for them occasions on weekends when you go to the beach or parties!

These days, it seems like everyone is talking about the ketogenic (in short, keto) diet - the very low-carbohydrate, moderate protein, high-fat eating plan that transforms your body into a fat-burning machine. Hollywood stars and professional athletes have publicly touted this diet's benefits, from losing weight, lowering blood sugar, fighting inflammation, reducing cancer risk, increasing energy, to slowing down aging. So is keto something that you should consider taking on? The following will explain what this diet is all about, the pros and cons, as well as the problems to look out for.

What Is Keto?

Normally, the body uses glucose as the main source of fuel for energy. When you are on a keto diet and you are eating very few carbs with only moderate amounts of protein (excess protein can be converted to carbs), your body switches its fuel supply to run mostly on fat. The liver produces ketones (a type of fatty acid) from fat. These ketones become a fuel source for the body, especially the brain which consumes plenty of energy and can run on either glucose or ketones.

When the body produces ketones, it enters a metabolic state called ketosis. Fasting is the easiest way to achieve ketosis. When you are fasting or eating very few carbs and only moderate amounts of protein, your body turns to burning stored fat for fuel. That is why people tend to lose more weight on the keto diet.

Benefits Of The Keto Diet

The keto diet is not new. It started being used in the 1920s as a medical therapy to treat epilepsy in children, but when anti-epileptic drugs came to the market, the diet fell into obscurity until recently. Given its success in reducing the number of seizures in epileptic patients, more and more research is being done on the ability of the diet to treat a range of neurologic disorders and other types of chronic illnesses.

Neurodegenerative diseases. New research indicates the benefits of keto in Alzheimer's, Parkinson's, autism, and multiple sclerosis (MS). It may also be protective in traumatic brain injury and stroke. One theory for keto's neuroprotective effects is that the ketones produced during ketosis provide additional fuel to brain cells, which may help those cells resist the damage from inflammation caused by these diseases.

Obesity and weight loss. If you are trying to lose weight, the keto diet is very effective as it helps to access and shed your body fat. Constant hunger is the biggest issue when you try to lose weight. The keto diet helps avoid this problem because reducing carb consumption and increasing fat intake promote satiety, making it easier for people to adhere to the diet. In a study, obese test subjects lost double the amount of weight within 24 weeks going on a low-carb diet (20.7 lbs) compared to the group on a low-fat diet (10.5 lbs).

Type 2 diabetes. Apart from weight loss, the keto diet also helps enhance insulin sensitivity, which is ideal for anyone with type 2 diabetes. In a study published in Nutrition & Metabolism, researchers noted that diabetics who ate low-carb keto diets were able to significantly reduce their dependence on diabetes medication and may even reverse it eventually. Additionally, it improves other health markers such as lowering triglyceride and LDL (bad) cholesterol and raising HDL (good) cholesterol.

Cancer. Most people are not aware that cancer cells' main fuel is glucose. That means eating the right diet may help suppress cancer growth. Since the keto diet is very low in carbs, it deprives the cancer cells of their primary source of fuel, which is sugar. When the body produces ketones, the healthy cells can use that as energy but not the cancer cells, so they are effectively being starved to death. As early as 1987, studies on keto diets have already demonstrated reduced tumor growth and improved survival for a number of cancers.

Comparing Standard American, Paleo, & Keto Diets

(As a % of total caloric intake)

____Carbs_______________Protein____
_________Fat

Standard   American   Diet_______40-60%______________15-30%_____________15-40%

Paleo   Diet_____________________________20-40%_____________20-35%_____________25-50%

Keo   Diet_________________________   ___5-10%______________10-15%_____________70-80%

The key distinction between the keto diet and the standard American or Paleo diets is that it contains far fewer carbs and much more fat. The keto diet results in ketosis with circulating ketones ranging from 0.5-5.0 mM. This can be measured using a home blood ketone monitor with ketone test strips. (Please know that testing ketones in urine is not accurate.)

How To Formulate A Keto Diet

1. Carbohydrates

For most people, to achieve ketosis (getting ketones above 0.5 mM) requires them to restrict carbs to somewhere between 20-50 grams (g)/day. The actual amount of carbs will vary from person to person. Generally, the more insulin resistant a person is, the more resistant they are to ketosis. Some insulin sensitive athletes exercising vigorously can consume more than 50 g/day and remain in ketosis, whereas individuals with type 2 diabetes and insulin resistance may need to be closer to 20-30 g/day.

When calculating carbs, one is allowed to use net carbs, meaning total carbs minus fiber and sugar alcohols. The concept of net carbs is to incorporate only carbs that increase blood sugar and insulin. Fiber does not have any metabolic or hormonal impact and so do most sugar alcohols. The exception is maltitol, which can have a non-trivial impact on blood sugar and insulin. Therefore, if maltitol is on the ingredient list, sugar alcohol should not be deducted from total carbs.

The level of carbs one can consume and remain in ketosis may also change over time depending on keto adaptation, weight loss, exercise habits, medications, etc. Therefore, one should measure his/her ketone levels on a routine basis.

In terms of the overall diet, carb-dense foods like pastas, cereals, potatoes, rice, beans, sugary sweets, sodas, juices, and beer are not suitable.

Most dairy products contain carbs in the form of lactose (milk sugar). However, some have less carbs and can be used regularly. These include hard cheeses (Parmesan, cheddar), soft, high-fat cheeses (Brie), full-fat cream cheese, heavy whipping cream, and sour cream.

A carb level less than 50 g/day generally breaks down to the following:

- 5-10 g carbs from protein-based foods. Eggs, cheese, and shellfish will carry a few residual grams of carbs from natural sources and added marinades and spices.
- 10-15 g carbs from non-starchy vegetables.

- 5-10 g carbs from nuts/seeds. Most nuts contain 5-6 g carbs per ounce.

- 5-10 g carbs from fruits such as berries, olives, tomatoes, and avocados.

- 5-10 g carbs from miscellaneous sources such as low-carb desserts, high-fat dressings, or drinks with very small amounts of sugar.

Beverages

Most people require at least half a gallon of total fluid per day. The best sources are filtered water, organic coffee and tea (regular and decaf, unsweetened), and unsweetened almond and coconut milk. Diet sodas and drinks are best avoided as they contain artificial sweeteners. If you drink red or white wine, limit to 1-2 glasses, the dryer the better. If you drink spirits, avoid the sweetened mixed drinks.

2. Protein

A keto diet is not a high protein diet. The reason is that protein increases insulin and can be converted to glucose through a process called gluconeogenesis, hence, inhibiting ketosis. However, a keto diet should not be too low in protein either as it can lead to loss of muscle tissue and function.

The average adult requires about 0.8-1.5 g per kilogram (kg) of lean body mass per day. It is important to make the calculation based on lean body mass, not total body weight. The reason is because fat mass does not re□uire protein to maintain, only the lean muscle mass.

For example, if an individual weighs 150 lbs (or 150/2.2 = 68.18 kg) and has a body fat content of 20% (or lean body mass of 80% = 68.18 kg x 0.8 = 54.55 kg), the protein requirement may range from 44 (= 54.55 x 0.8) to 82 (= 54.55 x 1.5) g/day.

Those who are insulin resistant or doing the keto diet for therapeutic reasons (cancer, epilepsy, etc.) should aim to be closer to the lower protein limit. The higher limit is for those who are very active or athletic. For everyone else who is using the keto diet for weight loss or other health benefits, the amount of daily protein can be somewhere in between.

Best sources of high quality protein include:

- Organic, pastured eggs (6-8 g of protein/egg)
- Grass-fed meats (6-9 g of protein/oz)
- Animal-based sources of omega-3 fats, such as wild-caught Alaskan salmon, sardines, and anchovies, and herrings. (6-9 g of protein/oz)
- Nuts and seeds, such as macadamia, almonds, pecans, flax, hemp, and sesame seeds. (4-8 g of protein/quarter cup)
- Vegetables (1-2 g of protein/oz)

3. Fat

Having figured out the exact amounts of carbs and protein to eat, the rest of the diet comes from fat. A keto diet is necessarily high in fat. If sufficient fat is eaten, body weight is maintained. If weigh loss is desired, one should consume less dietary fat and rely on stored body fat for energy expenditure instead.

(As a % of total caloric intake)

_______________________________________Maintain   Weight_________Lose Weight

Carbs_______________________________5-10%_______________________________5-10%

Protein_______________________________10-15%_______________________________10-15%

Fat from diet_______________________70-80%_______________________________35-40%

Fat from stored body fat_____0%_______________________________35-40%

For individuals who consume 2,000 calories a day to maintain their weight, daily fat intakes range from about 156-178 g/day. For large or very active individuals with high energy requirements who are maintaining weight, fat intakes may even exceed 300 g/day.

Most people can tolerate high intakes of fat, but certain conditions such as gallbladder removal may affect the amount of fat that can be consumed at a single meal. In which case, more frequent meals or use of bile salts or pancreatic enzymes high in lipase may be helpful.

Avoid eating undesirable fats such as trans fat, highly refined polyunsaturated vegetable oils, as well as high amounts of omega-6 polyunsaturated fats.

Best foods to obtain high quality fats include:

- Avocados and avocado oil
- Coconuts and coconut oil
- Grass-fed butter, ghee, and beef fat
- Organic, pastured heavy cream
- Olive oil
- Lard from pastured pigs
- Medium chain triglycerides (MCTs)

MCT is a specific type of fat that is metabolized differently from regular long-chain fatty acids. The liver can use MCTs to rapidly produce energy, even before glucose, thus allowing an increased production of ketones.

Concentrated sources of MCT oil are available as supplements. Many people use them to help achieve ketosis. The only food that is uniquely high in MCTs is coconut oil. About two-thirds of the coconut fat is derived from MCT.

Who Should Be Cautious With A Keto Diet?

For most people, a keto diet is very safe. However, there are certain individuals who need to take special care and discuss with their doctors before going on such a diet.

- Those taking medications for diabetes. Dosage may need to be adjusted as blood sugar goes down with a low-carb diet.
- Those taking medications for high blood pressure. Dosage may need to be adjusted as blood pressure goes down with a low-carb diet.
- Those who are breastfeeding should not go on a very strict low-carb diet as the body can lose about 30 g of carbs per day via the milk. Therefore, have at least 50 g of carbs per day while breastfeeding.
- Those with kidney disease should consult with their doctors before doing a keto diet.

Common Concerns With A Keto Diet

Not being able to reach ketosis. Make sure you are not eating too much protein and there is no hidden carbs in the packaged foods that you consume.

Eating the wrong kinds of fat such as the highly refined polyunsaturated corn and soybean oils.

Symptoms of a "keto-flu", such as feeling light-headed, dizziness, headaches, fatigue, brain fog, and constipation. When in ketosis, the body tends to excrete more sodium. If one is not getting enough sodium from the diet, symptoms of a keto-flu may appear. This is easily remedied by drinking 2 cups of broth (with added salt) per day. If you exercise vigorously or the sweat rate is high, you may need to add back even more sodium.

Dawn effect. Normal fasting blood sugars are less than 100 mg/dl and most people in ketosis will achieve this level if they are not diabetic. However, in some people fasting blood sugars tend to increase, especially in the morning, while on a keto diet. This is called the "dawn effect" and is due to the normal circadian rise in morning cortisol (stress hormone) that stimulates the liver to make more glucose. If this happens, make sure you are not consuming excessive protein at dinner and not too close to bedtime. Stress and poor sleep can also lead to higher cortisol levels. If you are insulin resistant, you may also need more time to achieve ketosis.

Low athletic performance. Keto-adaptation usually takes about 4 weeks. During which, instead of doing intense workouts or training, switch to something that is less vigorous. After the adaptation period, athletic performance usually returns to normal or even better, especially for endurance sports.

Keto-rash is not a common side effect of the diet. Probable causes include production of acetone (a form of ketone) in the sweat that irritates the skin or nutrient deficiencies including protein or minerals. Shower immediately after exercise and make sure you eat nutrient dense whole foods.

Ketoacidosis. This is a very rare condition that occurs when blood ketone levels go above 15 mM. A well-formulated keto diet does not cause ketoacidosis. Certain conditions such as type 1 diabetes, being on medications with SGLT-2 inhibitors for type 2 diabetes, or breastfeeding re□uire extra caution. Symptoms include lethargy, nausea, vomiting, and rapid shallow breathing. Mild cases can be resolved using sodium bicarbonate mixed with diluted orange or apple juice. Severe symptoms re□uire prompt medical attention.

Is Keto Safe For Long-Term?

This is an area of some controversy. Though there have not been any studies indicating any adverse long-term effects of being on a keto diet, many experts now believe that the body may develop a "resistance" to the benefits of ketosis unless one regularly cycles in and out of it. In addition, eating a very high-fat diet in the long-term may not be suitable for all body types.

Cyclical keto diet

Once you are able to generate over 0.5 mM of ketones in the blood on a consistent basis, it is time to start reintroducing carbs back into the diet. Instead of eating merely 20-50 g of carbs/day, you may want to increase it to 100-150 g on those carb-feeding days. Typically, 2-3 times a week will be sufficient. Ideally, this is also done on strength training days on which you actually increase your protein intake.

This approach of cycling may make the diet plan more acceptable to some people who are reluctant to permanently eliminate some of their favorite foods. However, it may also lower resolve and commitment to the keto diet or trigger binges in susceptible individuals.

IS THE KETO DIET RIGHT FOR YOU?

Are you interested in losing weight? Are you tired of diets that advocate low or no fats and crave your high fat meats? You may well be considering going on the keto diet, the new kid on the block. Endorsed by many celebrities including Halle Berry, LeBron James and Kim Kardashian among others, the keto diet has been the subject of much debate among dietitians and doctors. Do you wonder if the keto diet is safe and right for you?

What is the ketogenic diet anyway?

You must be aware that the body uses sugar in the form of glycogen to function. The keto diet that is extremely restricted in sugar forces your body to use fat as fuel instead of sugar, since it does not get enough sugar. When the body does not get enough sugar for fuel, the liver is forced to turn the available fat into ketones that are used by the body as fuel - hence the term ketogenic.

This diet is a high fat diet with moderate amounts of protein. Depending on your carb intake the body reaches a state of ketosis in less than a week and stays there. As fat is used instead of sugar for fuel in the body, the weight loss is dramatic without any supposed restriction of calories.

The keto diet is such that it you should aim to get 60-75% of your daily calories from fat, 15-30% from protein and only 5-10% from carbohydrates. This usually means that you can eat only 20-50 grams of carbs in a day.

What can you eat on this diet?

The diet is a high fat diet that is somewhat similar to Atkins. However, there is greater emphasis on fats, usually 'good' fats. On the keto diet you can have

- Olive oil
- Coconut oil
- Nut oils
- Butter
- Ghee
- Grass fed beef
- Chicken
- Fish
- Other meats
- Full fat cheese
- Eggs
- Cream
- Leafy greens
- Non-starchy vegetables

- Nuts
- Seeds

You can also get a whole range of snacks that are meant for keto followers. As you can see from this list, fruits are restricted. You can have low sugar fruits in a limited quantity (mostly berries), but will have to forego your favorite fruits as these are all sweet and/or starchy.

This diet includes no grains of any kind, starchy vegetables like potatoes (and all tubers), no sugar or sweets, no breads and cakes, no beans and lentils, no pasta, no pizza and burgers and very little alcohol. This also means no coffee with milk or tea with milk - in fact, no milk and ice-creams and milk based desserts.

Many of these have workarounds as you can get carbohydrate free pasta and pizza, you can have cauliflower rice and now there are even restaurants that cater to keto aficionados.

What are the benefits of the keto diet?

If you are wondering if this diet is safe, its proponents and those who have achieved their weight loss goals will certainly agree that it is safe. Among the benefits of the keto diet you can expect:

- Loss of weight
- Reduced or no sugar spikes
- Appetite control
- Seizure controlling effect
- Blood pressure normalizes in high blood pressure patients
- Reduced attacks of migraine
- Type 2 diabetes patients on this diet may be able to reduce their medications

Some benefits to those suffering from cancer

Apart from the first four, there is not sufficient evidence to support its effectiveness or otherwise for other diseases as a lot more research is required over the long-term.

Are there any side-effects of this diet?

When you initially start the keto diet, you can suffer from what is known as keto flu. These symptoms may not occur in all people and usually start a few days after being on the diet, when your body is in a state of ketosis. Some of the side-effects are:

- Nausea
- Cramps and tummy pain
- Headache
- Vomiting
- Diarrhea and/or constipation
- Muscle cramps
- Dizziness and poor concentrations
- Insomnia
- Carbohydrate and sugar cravings

These may take up to a week to subside as your body get used to the new diet regime. You can also suffer from other problems when you start the keto diet - you may find that you have increased urination, so it is important to keep yourself well hydrated. You may also suffer from keto breath when your body reaches optimal ketosis and you can use a mouthwash or brush your teeth more frequently.

Usually the side effects are temporary and once your body acclimatizes to the new diet, these should disappear.

How safe is the keto diet?

Just like any other diet that restricts foods in specific categories, the keto diet is not without risks. As you are not supposed to eat many fruits and vegetables, beans and lentils and other foods, you can suffer from lack of many essential nutrients. Since the diet is high in saturated fats and, if you indulge in the 'bad' fats, you can have high cholesterol levels upping your risk of heart disease.

In the long-term the keto diet can also cause many nutritional deficiencies since you cannot eat grains, many fruits and vegetables and miss out on fiber as also important vitamins, minerals, phytonutrients and antioxidants among other things. You can suffer from gastrointestinal distress, lowered bone density (no dairy and other sources of calcium) and kidney and liver problems (the diet puts added stress on both the organs).

Is the keto diet safe for you?

If you are willing to forego your usual dietary staples and are really keen to lose weight, you may be tempted to try out the keto diet. The biggest issue with this diet is poor patient compliance thanks to the carbohydrate restriction, so you have to be sure that you can live with your food choices. If you simply find it too difficult to follow, you can go on a version of the modified keto diet that offers more carbs.

However, the keto diet is definitely effective in helping you lose weight. According to a recent study many of the obese patients followed were successful in losing weight. Any problems that they faced were temporary. If you do not have any significant health problems except for obesity and have been unsuccessful in losing weight following any conventional diet, the keto diet may a viable option. You must be absolutely determined to lose the weight and be prepared to go on a restricted diet as specified. Even if you have any medical problems, you can take your doctor's advice and a nutritionist's guidance and go on this diet.

Another study that was carried out for a longer time showed that going on the keto diet is beneficial in weight loss and also results in reduced cholesterol levels with a decrease in the bad cholesterol and an increase in the good cholesterol.

Is the keto diet safe for you? Most doctors and nutritionists are agreed that the keto diet is good for weight loss over the short-term. As for the long-term, more studies are needed. Do keep in mind that obesity is not an apt choice as it comes with its own risk of health problems.

SHOULD WOMEN AVOID THE KETO DIET?

The Keto Diet has become Quite a popular topic in the fitness community. It has been found to aid in the loss of weight and lowering the inflammation in the gut. New research has shown positive effects for both men and women adhering to a keto style diet.

What is the Keto Diet?

First, a keto, or ketogenic diet, is designed to keep your body in more of a ketosis state. Ketosis is not abnormal. It is a state where your body is low on carbohydrate fuel. When this occurs, it starts to burn fat, rather than the carbs. The process produces ketones. The average person does not stay in a ketogenic state except during heavy exercise, such as CrossFit, or during pregnancy.

A ketogenic diet promotes very low carbohydrate and higher fat intake. The body will in turn, use fat to produce energy. This diet has also been shown to decrease autoimmune diseases, endocrine diseases, and also has cancer fighting properties.

Ketosis can be an issue with diabetics. This can occur if not using enough insulin.

How does Keto benefit CrossFit athletes?

As stated earlier, a ketogenic diet helps to burn fat, thus losing weight. This low carb diet is similar to the Paleo Diet. We are a strong proponent of Paleo because it promotes higher protein for fuel instead of carbs. As we stated earlier, the keto diet uses fat rather than protein for fuel. A keto and paleo diet both burn fat while maintaining muscle.

An athlete exercising at a high level, such as CrossFit, will see increased energy and fat loss, without decreasing muscle mass.

Why is the Keto Diet good for women?

The benefits of being a woman on this diet are surprisingly good. In addition to the weight loss and muscle gain, a keto diet has an amazing way of helping the endocrine system. We all realize the effect hormones have on the woman athlete.

Fluctuating hormones can cause pain, fatigue, and even depression. The link between hormones and cancer cannot be denied. A keto diet has shown to better regulate the endocrine system. By doing this, it decreases the incidence of some cancers, thyroid disease, and diabetes.

How does a women initiate a keto diet?

Slowly and carefully. A keotgenic diet should not be started at a full 100 percent. You should slowly decrease the amount of carbs you consume. Cutting the carbs too quickly can actually have a negative effect. It can stress the body and confuse it, thus causing a wild imbalance.

Also, if pregnant or nursing, you should not use a keto diet. During this period, eat a well-rounded diet of fruits, vegetables, dairy, and grains.

My best advice, get your body as stable as possible, and then slowly incorporate a ketogenic diet.

The ketogenic diet, colloquially called the keto diet, is a popular diet containing high amounts of fats, adequate protein and low carbohydrate. It is also referred to as a Low Carb-High Fat (LCHF) diet and a low carbohydrate diet.

Ketogenic diets are basically designed to induce a state of ketosis in the body. When the amount of glucose in the body becomes too low, the body switches to fat as an alternative source of energy.

The body has two primary fuel sources which are:

- glucose
- free fatty acids (FFA) and, to a lesser extent, ketones made from FFA

Fat deposits are stored in the form of triglycerides. They are normally broken down into long-chain fatty acids and glycerol. Stripping off the glycerol from the triglyceride molecule allows for the release of the three free fatty acid (FFA) molecules into the bloodstream to be used as energy.

The glycerol molecule goes into the liver where three molecules of it combine to form one glucose molecule. Therefore, as your body burns fat, it also produces glucose as a by-product. This glucose can be used to fuel parts of the brain as well as other parts of the body that cannot run on FFA.

However, while glucose can travel through the bloodstream on its own, cholesterol and triglycerides need a carrier to move around in the bloodstream. Cholesterol and triglycerides are packaged in a carrier called low-density lipoprotein, or LDL. Thus, the larger the LDL particle, the more triglycerides it contains.

The overall process of burning fat deposits for energy produces carbon dioxide, water, and compounds called ketones.

Ketones are produced by the liver from free fatty acids. There are composed of 2 groups of atoms linked together by a carbonyl functional group.

The body has no capability to store ketones and therefore they must be either used or excreted. The body excrete them either through the breath as acetone or through the urine as acetoacetate.

Ketones can be used by body cells as a source of energy. Also, the brain can make use of ketones in generating about 70-75% of its energy requirement.

Like alcohol, ketones take priority as a fuel source over carbohydrates. This implies that when they are high in the bloodstream, they must be burned first before glucose can be used as a fuel.

What Causes Ketosis

When you start eating less amounts of carbohydrates, your body gets smaller supply of glucose to use as energy compared to before.

The decrease in the amount of consumed carbohydrates and the subsequent reduction in the amount of available glucose, slowly forces the body to move into the state of ketosis. Thus, the body goes into a state of ketosis when there is not enough amount of glucose available to the body cells.

Starvation Induced Ketosis

Fasting and starvation states usually involve reduced or no intake of food that the body can digest and convert into glucose. While starvation is involuntary, fasting is a more conscious choice you make to intentionally not eat.

However, the body enters into a "starvation mode" whenever you are sleeping, when you skip a meal or when you intentionally go on a fast. The lack of food intake results in a reduction in blood glucose levels. As a result, the body starts to break down it glycogen (stored glucose) stores for energy.

The glycogen is converted back into glucose and used as energy by the body. In this state, the body also starts to burn its stored fats. Thus, the production of ketone bodies (ketogenesis) is induced by a lack of available glucose.

Any time the amount of ketones in the blood outnumber the molecules of glucose, the body cells will start making use of the ketones as their source of energy.

You've probably heard plenty about the Atkins Diet over the years. You know, that incredibly popular and controversial diet that involves cutting right down on your carbohydrate intake. You may have also heard of "ketogenic diets" - it's a more scientific term so you may not recognise it. Did you realise that the Atkins Diet is a type of ketogenic diet? In this article we'll have a brief look at what the term means and my experience of this type of diet.

The Atkins Diet

The original Atkins Diet book, Dr. Atkins' Diet Revolution, was released in 1972. Dr Robert Atkins was interested, among other things, in getting his own weight under control. Primarily using self-experimentation techniques he found that eating a diet very low in carbohydrates tended to make him lose weight quickly. His experimentation was based upon other research papers and, as a result of his own studies, he became confident that the science behind the diet was sound. The resulting book was a resounding success and, over the next 30 years up to his death in 2003, Robert Atkins continued to produce popular diet books based upon the low-carbohydrate principle.

Ketogenic Diets

Some would argue that only the first "phase" of the Atkins Diet is "ketogenic" but it's very clear that this element is central to the whole diet. There are many other diets of this type with different names and claims but, if they talk about severely restricting the intake of carbohydrates, then they're probably forms of ketogenic diet. The process of "ketosis" is □uite complicated and would take some time to describe but, in essence, it works because cutting down on carbs restricts the amount of blood glucose available to trigger the "insulin response". Without a triggering of the glucose-insulin response some hormonal changes take place which cause the body to start burning its stores of fat as energy. This also has the interesting effect of causing your brain to be fuelled by what are known as "ketone bodies" (hence "ketogenic") rather than the usual glucose. The whole process is really □uite fascinating and I recommend that you read up on it.

Controversy

All forms of ketogenic diet are controversial. Most of the debate surrounds the issue of cholesterol and whether ketogenic diets increase or decrease the levels HDL "good" cholesterol and/or increase or decrease LDL "bad" cholesterol. The number of scientific studies is increasing year on year and it is certainly possible to point to strong cases on both sides of the argument. My conclusion (and this is only my opinion) is that one could e□ually make the case that a carbohydrate-laden diet has negative effects on cholesterol and I think that, on balance, a ketogenic-type diet is more healthy than a carbohydrate-heavy one. Interestingly, there isn't so much controversy about whether ketogenic diets work or not (it's widely accepted that they do); it's mostly about how they work and whether that is good/bad/indifferent from a health perspective.

The KETO COOKBOOK is a MUST HAVE - an ABSOLUTE MUST HAVE - for all families, carers and associated professionals who need a thorough understanding of the Ketogenic Diet and it's application for helping reduce seizures in children with epilepsy, and some other neurological conditions.

The Keto Cookbook, co-authored by Dawn Martinez and Laura Cramp, RD, LD, CNSC, is written with the same precision and detail which the very nature of the diet dictates, reflecting the awareness, skills and extensive experience of both women.

Dawn is the mother of Charlotte, who has Dravet's Syndrome, and who has responded so successfully to the Keto Diet after exhaustive and unsuccessful attempts with AEDs anti epileptic drugs.

Laura is a specialist dietitian at The Children's National Medical Centre in Washington, DC, working not only with patients and their families, but advising medical professionals and hospital food staff on the intricacies of using the Ketogenic Diet to treat epilepsy and reduce seizures.

Gone is the myth that this diet is unappetizing, unpalatable, boring and unappealing ! Beautifully illustrated recipes for 96 different delicious meals and snacks are testimony to this. All recipes:

- are Keto approved

- give the calorie count

- give exact ingredients for a 4:1 ratio diet

- are further described with symbols denoting other aspects of the recipe, e.g. " Quick", " "Vegetarian", "Freezes well".

The actual diet, though all important, is only one of many aspects Keto families need to address and fully understand.

Other chapters covering all contingencies to make the rigorous demands of the Ketogenic Diet as manageable as possible include:

- stocking the pantry for the emergencies presented both by unanticipated calamities of the daily schedule to major emergencies such as power-outs, flood, being snowbound etc.

- keeping a supply of instant snacks and frozen meals which can be quickly...

- presentation of the kitchen by removing any temptations from prying fingers

- e□uipping the kitchen with the essentials for meal preparation, to cut time without precision

- sample letters to present at airports, schools, hospitals etc to facilitate the situation

I highly recommend the "Keto Cookbook" because in the world of the Ketogenic diet, it would be hard to match the combined knowledge and experience of the authors, who have written precisely and professionally, but from a base of heartache and love.

It is hard to estimate the happiness brought to a family of a child suffering with uncontrollable seizures when the Keto Diet is successful in reducing or eliminating seizures. From watching helplessly as their child slowly deteriorates and slips behind developmentally, to seeing the success of the diet the child re-emerging with their previously known personal, developmentally progressing, regaining speech and other important milestones is an unimaginable stress replaced with unimaginable joy for those involved.

THE BENEFITS OF MIXING MCT OIL INTO YOUR KETOGENIC DIET PLAN

In life, we're always talking about must haves. If you're driving a high end car, you must have the top of the line motor oil coursing through its cylinders. If you're competing at a high level in a track competition, state of the art running shoes are a must have. When you're celebrating a huge quarter at the office, the finest bourbon is a must have. I would submit to you, that if you're serious about a ketogenic lifestyle, MCT Oil is a must have.

MCT Oil provides a heavy dose of the very fuels that turn your body into - and keep it - a fat burning machine. Unlike LCTs, MCTs bypass much of the digestion process that others fats go through. MCTs act in an almost carb-like manner in how they're sent directly to the liver, where they are used for energy.

There are many reasons why MCT makes perfect sense for your Ketogenic Diet, but help you understand how they can play an essential role in your nutrition, we've some of the main benefits of MCT Oil in your Ketogenic Diet plan.

MCT OIL HELPS YOUR GET INTO KETOSIS FASTER

As you already know, MCTs go to your liver, and act in a "carb-like" manner that LCTs do not have the ability to do. This means that you can theoretically kickstart Ketosis by following these steps:

1. Fast with no breakFAST.

If you've been out of Ketosis for awhile and you want to efficiently get back into a fat burning state, a mix of fasting and MCT Oil will do the job. Just eat a very low carb dinner, or even skip dinner, and then wake up and don't eat breakfast! Instead, drink a cup of coffee, and put a tablespoon or two of MCT Oil into your coffee and head out!

The shot of MCT, plus the already fasted state of your body will have you back into Ketosis quicker than if you tried to just slowly eat your way back into Ketosis (i.e. nutritional Ketosis). It's also worth adding that the energy you get from the MCT Oil and the coffee will be unlike what you were used to: the MCTs provide a prolonged energy that isn't comparable to energy derived from glycogen.

2. Meal replacement with MCT Oil

Another benefit that comes from using MCT Oil in your Ketogenic Diet plan is using it as a meal replacement.

This somewhat resembles the previous point of fasting with MCT Oil, but the difference is that you're still eating other regular Ketogenic meals, except your replacing (at least) one of those meals with some MCT Oil.

One of the benefits of MCT Oil is its ability to satiate your appetite. So while it sounds initially scary to just depend a few tablespoons of oil for a meal replacement, your body will become accustomed as you do it more and more. The MCTs will act as replacement for what's normally there (glycogen) and your fierce-badger-hunger cravings will lessen.

In our fast paced, 21st century lifestyle, the benefits of being able to remain in Ketosis while only slurping a few tablespoons of MCTs cannot be overstated.

3. Ramp up your Ketogenic dishes with MCT

MCT Oil's versatility is amazing. Let's say you're already in Ketosis, but you're about to eat a salad for your daily carbs, and you want to keep it 100 on the Keto life. It's easy! Just use MCT for a base to your dressing, and you can rest assured that you'll still be burning fat after you've downed your greens!

Another way to use MCTs in your favorite Ketogenic meals is to use it as a replacement for regular oil in baking! There's a whole ocean of Keto baking recipes out there, so why not double down and use MCT instead of regular coconut oil?!

But what if you're not baking? What if you're out for a jog and you want to implement the energy efficiency of MCT Oil? How about a nice Keto "sports drink"?! All you have to do is it to water, and then squeeze in some lemon juice, and you'll have a healthier, non-sugary sports drink for long workouts in the sun!

There are many ways to skin a cat, and there's also many ways to amplify your Ketogenic Diet. MCTs are essential to your body transforming into a fat burning machine. Unfortunately, you're not always going to be able to get the proper amounts from a diet alone - you'll need a boost, and MCT Oil is that boost.

Life is full of "must haves," and your diet does not fall out of the realm of this mantra. If you want to live a truly Ketogenic lifestyle, you're going to have invest in the right fuels, and implement them in the most efficient ways possible. So what's the benefit of MCT to your Ketogenic Diet plan? The answer: efficiency. An efficient diet, which feeds an efficient lifestyle, that ultimately gives you more time to do the things you love.

Keto breakfasts don't have to be the same old bacon and eggs every single day. There are endless ways to create nourishing meals that are high fat, low carb and have a boost of protein. Luckily, we did the work for you and found the tastiest keto breakfast recipes. The best part? They're filled with nourishing, Paleo-approved ingredients, too!

Even if you're not keto, these low-carb keto breakfast recipes are rich in healthy fats and proteins that will promote blood sugar balance, weight loss, and long-term satiety to finally end those late morning hungry feelings that attack before lunch.

1. <u>Keto Breakfast Burger with Avocado Buns</u>

You'll get your fingers messy eating this one, but it's well worth it. Never have avocado, egg, or bacon been paired quite so perfectly.

This low-carb, high-fat recipe swaps the classic burger bun with two halves of an avocado, resulting in a ketogenic food lovers' dream. Then to top it all off, crispy bacon and a fried egg are added.

To start, slice the avocados in half width-wise. Remove the pit and scoop the avocado out of its skin. Begin building your burger by adding the toppings of your choice and finish with a dollop of Paleo mayo or a slice of cashew cheese. Don't forget to sprinkle some sesame seeds on top!

Ingredients:

- 1 ripe avocado
- 1 egg
- 2 bacon rashers
- 1 red onion slice
- 1 tomato slice
- 1 lettuce leaf
- 1 T Paleo mayonnaise
- Sea salt, to taste
- Sesame seeds, for garnish

Instructions:

1. Place the bacon rashers on a cold frying pan. Turn the stove on and start frying the bacon. When bacon beings to curl, flip it with a fork. Continue cooking the bacon until it is crispy.

2. Remove the bacon from the pan and crack the egg into the same pan, using the bacon fat to cook it. Cook until the white is set but the yolk is still runny.

3. Slice the avocados in half width-wise. Remove the pit and use a spoon to scoop it out of its skin.

4. Fill the hole where the pit used to be with Paleo mayonnaise.

5. Layer with lettuce, tomato, onion, bacon, and fried egg.

6. Season with sea salt.

7. Top with the second half of the avocado.

8. Sprinkle with sesame seeds.

2. Creamy Cauliflower and Ground Beef Skillet

Want proof that ground beef isn't just for dinner? This one-pan recipe nestles eggs into a skillet of beef and cauliflower and sprinkled with avocado for a hunger-stomping brekkie.

Ingredients:

- 2 tsbp ghee (or make your own)
- ½ small onion, chopped
- 2 cloves garlic, chopped
- 4 jalapeño peppers, sliced

- 454g (1lb) lean ground beef
- 1 tsp Himalayan salt
- ½ tsp freshly cracked black pepper
- 1 small head cauliflower (454g | 1lb), grated
- ½ cup paleo mayo
- ½ cup water
- ¼ cup toasted sunflower seed butter
- 1 tbsp coconut aminos
- 1 tsp fish sauce
- 1 tsp ground cumin
- 4 large eggs
- 2 jalapeño peppers, sliced
- ½ ripe avocado, diced
- 2 tbsp paleo mayo
- 1 tbsp apple cider vinegar
- 1 tbsp fresh parsley, chopped

Instructions:

1. Melt ghee in a heavy skillet (cast iron preferred) set over medium-high heat. When the fat is nice and hot, add onion, garlic and jalapeño pepper and cook until fragrant and softened, about 2-3 minutes.

2. Add ground beef, salt and pepper and continue cooking until the beef is completely brown. Lower the heat to medium-low and throw in the grated cauliflower; stir well and continue

cooking for 2-3 minutes. (You can use a box grater or the grater disc of your food processor to grate the cauliflower.)

3. Meanwhile, add the mayo, water, sunflower seed butter, coconut aminos, fish sauce and cumin to a large measuring cup and whisk until well combined.

4. Pour that over the ground beef and cauliflower mixture and stir until well incorporated. Continue cooking for about 3-5 minutes, until all the li□uid has been absorbed.

5. Remove from heat, spread the meat mixture nice and evenly and make 4 shallow dimples on top. Crack one egg in each of the dimples then sprinkle with salt and pepper and sliced jalapeño peppers.

6. Set your oven to broil and place the skillet right under the broiler for about 8-10 minutes or until the eggs are cooked to your liking.

7. In the meantime, mix 2 tablespoons of mayo with the apple cider vinegar.

8. Drizzle all over the skillet as soon as it comes out of the oven, then garnish with diced avocado and fresh chopped parsley.

9. Poke the yolks and serve immediately.

3. Breakfast BLT Salad

This one-dish breakfast is low prep and high on nutrients. Don't have kale? Baby spinach works just as well. Salad for breakfast? Yes!! This

Breakfast BLT Salad can be eaten anytime of the day really, but eggs and bacon served over this simple massaged kale salad with avocado and tomatoes is a delicious, savory, healthy breakfast idea.

Ingredients:

- 3 cups shredded Lacinto kale, no stems
- 1 teaspoon red wine vinegar
- 2 teaspoons extra virgin olive oil
- kosher salt
- black pepper, to taste
- 2 large eggs
- 4 strips cooked center cut bacon, chopped
- 2 ounces sliced avocado
- 10 grape tomatoes, halved

Instructions:

1. In a bowl combine the kale, olive oil, vinegar and 1/4 teaspoon salt. Massage with your hands for about 3 minutes, until the kale softens.
2. Cook eggs to desired likeness, I prefer them soft boiled. How to Make Perfect Eggs in the Instant Pot.

3. Divide the kale between two bowls, top with bacon, tomatoes, avocado and egg.

4. Finish with pinch of salt and pepper.

4. Cheesy Broccoli Breakfast Muffins

Cheesy yet dairy-free, these broccoli muffins prep fast and make a perfect on-the-go breakfast. Each muffin is just 5 net carbs, so go ahead and have two!

These warm, grain-free treats taste like broccoli cheddar soup in a muffin!

Tools

- Muffin tin
- Mixing bowl

Ingredients:

- 2 t ghee, softened + extra for greasing

- 1 cup broccoli florets, finely chopped
- 2 cups almond flour
- 2 large pasture-raised eggs
- 1 cup unsweetened almond milk
- 2 T nutritional yeast
- 1 t baking powder
- 1/2 t sea salt

Instructions:

1. Preheat the oven to 350°F and grease a large muffin tin with ghee.
2. Stir together all the ingredients in a large mixing bowl until well combined.
3. Spoon the mixture into the muffin tins. Bake for 30 minutes until a toothpick inserted in the center comes out clean.

5. Paleo Breakfast Pizza

Even with the crust, this pizza dish is perfectly keto. Customize it with your favorite keto toppings to make any meal pizza night.

Ingredients:

For the crust:

- 6 large egg whites
- 1/2 cup coconut flour
- 1 cup coconut milk unsweetened
- 1 tsp onion powder
- 2 tsp garlic powder
- 2 tsp Italian seasoning
- 1/2 tsp baking soda

For the toppings:

- 3 large eggs
- 1 tomato thinly sliced
- 1 cup baby spinach
- 1/2 tsp red pepper flakes
- 1 tbsp extra virgin olive oil

Instructions:

1. Preheat the oven to 375 degrees F. Prepare a large baking sheet with parchment paper.
2. In a large bowl, whisk together the egg whites, seasonings and coconut milk. Then fold in the coconut flour until combined.
3. Using a baking spatula, spread the dough onto the prepared baking sheet to form a rectangle.
4. Bake 15-18 minutes until the dough is set firmly.
5. Remove the crust from the oven and reduce the oven to 350 degrees F.
6. Using a baking brush or back of a spoon to spread the extra virgin olive oil over the crust. Spread the spinach over the crush, then the tomatoes. Carefully crack 3 eggs on top of the pizza. Sprinkle with the red pepper flakes.
7. Bake in the oven 12 minutes until the egg whites have set.
8. Remove from the oven and devour!

6. Hot and Crispy Cauliflower Fritters

Cauliflower is the most versatile keto-friendly ingredient that exists. If you hadn't made them yourself, you'd never know these fritters are low carb and loaded with veggies!

Serve up these warm, crispy cauliflower fritters morning, noon or night!

Tools

- Large pot
- Food processor
- Mixing bowl
- Spatula
- Large skillet

Ingredients:

- 1 large head of cauliflower, broken into florets
- 2 eggs
- 2/3 cup almond flour
- 1 T nutritional yeast
- 1/2 t turmeric
- 1/2 t sea salt
- 1/4 t black pepper
- 1-2 T ghee

Instructions:

1. Add the cauliflower to a large pot covered in water. Bring to a boil and boil for 8 minutes. Strain. Add the florets into a food processor and pulse until riced.
2. Add cauliflower, eggs, almond flour, nutritional yeast, turmeric, salt and pepper to a mixing bowl. Stir well to combine. Form into patties.
3. Heat the ghee over medium heat in a skillet. Scoop about half the mixture into three fritters and cook until golden brown on each side, 3-4 minutes. Set aside until the rest of the fritters are cooked. Serve hot.

7. Coconut Flour Porridge Breakfast Cereal

If you miss the convenience of a bowl of cereal for breakfast, you're in luck! This creamy, grain-free porridge is simple to throw together – just simmer everything together, and grab a spoon!

Ingredients:

- 2 tablespoons coconut flour
- 2 tablespoons golden flax meal
- 3/4 cup water
- pinch of salt

- 1 large egg, beaten
- 2 teaspoons butter or ghee
- 1 tablespoon heavy cream or coconut milk
- 1 tablespoon Sukrin Gold or your favorite sweetener

Instructions:

1. Measure the first four ingredients into a small pot over medium heat and stir. When it begins to simmer, turn it down to medium-low and whisk until it begins to thicken.
2. Remove the coconut flour porridge from heat and add the beaten egg, a half at a time, while whisking continuously. Place back on the heat and continue to whisk until the porridge thickens.
3. Remove from the heat and continue to whisk for about 30 seconds before adding the butter, cream and sweetener.
4. Garnish with your favorite toppings. (4 grams net carbs)

8. Spicy Shrimp Omelette

Jazz up plain eggs with this omelette filled with shrimp and spinach. No flipping or folding skills necessary!

Ingredients:

- 10 large shrimp
- 6 eggs
- 4 grape tomatoes
- 1 handful spinach
- 1/4 onion
- 1 tbsp sriracha salt
- 1 sprig parsley
- 1/4 tsp cayenne

Instructions:

1. Chop up some onion and slice the grape tomatoes in half lengthwise.
2. Fire up a pan to medium heat and throw on the onions and some salt to cook. At the same time, place the grape tomatoes cut side down to roast a little.
3. When the onions are translucent throw in your spinach and let it wilt and shrink enough for some shrimp to fit in.
4. Throw in the shrimp and move on to the eggs!

5. Here you have some flexibility: you can make a scramble (on low heat and stirring very often), or you can whisk the eggs in the bowl and pour it over to make a regular omelette. We decided to make a sunny side up omelette. You can also choose to crack the yolks after they're on the shrimp and spinach so you've got two layers of egg, making a nice marbled omelette.

6. To make the eggs our way, crack each one leaving room for all 6, or however many you're using. Then take a wooden spoon and jiggle the whites around so they grab everything underneath them a little better.

7. Put a lid on your pan so the top of your omelette cooks as well. We left ours on the fire for about 6-8 minutes. Watch you eggs, once a thin film of white is covering the yolks, it's ready. If you like your eggs less runny, cook it for a little longer than that.

8. When the omelette is done, run a knife across each yolk and let it ooze onto the entire omelette, adding new, yummy textures! Garnish with some parsley and enjoy!

9. White Chocolate Fat Bombs

It's the keto version of a white chocolate truffle, and it's the perfect way to start your morning. Enjoy it paired with bulletproof coffee or a nice cup of hot tea.

Ingredients:

- 1/4 cup cocoa butter about 25g
- 1/4 cup coconut oil about 35g

- 10 drops vanilla stevia drops

Instructions:

1. Melt together cocoa butter and coconut oil over low heat or in double boiler.
2. Remove from heat and stir in vanilla flavored stevia drops.
3. Pour into molds.
4. Chill until hardened.
5. Remove from molds and keep stored in the refrigerator.

Notes : Makes 8 fat bombs (1 tablespoon healthy oil each)

10. Egg Roll-Ups

Want something a little fancier than eggs in a pan? Try these magazine-worthy egg roll-ups. P.S. Don't forget to Instagram these so your keto buddies know your breakfast game is on point. The perfect brunch recipe or meal prep, you decide!

Scale

Ingredients:

- 10 large eggs
- 1/2 cup nut milk (I like my cashew cream or coconut milk)
- pinch of salt
- dash of pepper
- tsp of mustard
- 8 slices of bacon
- 1 cup chives
- 2 handfuls fresh, whole basil leaves
- 1 cup fresh arugula
- 1 ripe avocado
- 3 tbsp paleo mayo

Things You Will Need

- 1 half sized sheet pan with a 1 to a 2-inch rim (21x15in)

- a blender
- parchment paper
- coconut, avocado or another cooking spray, ideally.

Instructions:

1. Lay your bacon flat on a baking sheet, all in a row, the slices should not touch or overlap. Pop the sheet pan in the oven, middle rack. Set to 400F.
2. Once the oven reaches temp, check on the bacon, it will be par-cooked. Set a timer for 8-10 minutes. That should be enough time for it to cook up nice and crispy.
3. In the meantime, prep the rest of your ingredients. Crack the eggs into the blender. Add in the salt, pepper, milk, and mustard. Dice up chives. Get your basil leaves and arugula ready.
4. When the bacon is ready, remove from the oven. Use tongs to transfer the bacon to a cutting board. Don't turn off the oven!
5. Drain the fat from the sheet pan (to a jar, you better save that goodness).
6. Line that same sheet pan with parchment paper. Center it as much as possible so the sides reach the rim. Leave a little slack on either end so you can pull on it later. Then grease on the sheet pan will make it easy to flatten and smooth out the paper! Win!
7. Spray the top of the paper lightly with oil.

8. Crank that blender and whiz up the egg mix for 30 seconds.

9. Make sure your sheet pan in on an even, flat surface when you pour in the egg mix. If it's not settling evenly, help it out with a spatula.

10. Sprinkle the chives evenly all over your eggs.

11. Chop up the crispy bacon and sprinkle over the egg as well.

12. Bake for 20 minutes or until edges are golden and the center is completely set (it shouldn't jiggle at all).

13. Remove the sheet pan from the oven and let it cool for 10 minutes.

14. Check to see if your omelet is stuck to the parchment paper. If it's not, pick it up carefully and place it bottom side up on the cutting board.

15. If it is sticking to the parchment paper, then use the parchment paper to slide it onto the cutting board. Then flip it □uickly. Peel the parchment paper, starting on a corner and using your fingers to old the omelet down.

16. Once all the parchment paper has been removed, use a spatula to smear mayo all over this bad boy.

17. Starting about 2 inches from one end, let's say the left side, arrange your avocado slices in a vertical stripe. Next, the basil leaves and then the arugula, alternating until you have about an inch left.

18. Make sure your avocado is flat and there aren't any hard edges, for these could puncture your egg.

19. From the left side (where you have the two inches) gently pick it up and pull it over your avocado then fold in with your

fingers and begin to roll it as you would a burrito. If it tears a little at the sides in the first or second pass, don't worry, the outer layers will still hold it together.

20. Once you've rolled it up and have a massive egg log. Yes, it will be beastly! Slice it up. I like to cut it into 2-inch pieces.

21. Serve right away to a crowd or store in an airtight container for meal prep.

Notes: If you're making for meal prep, skip the avocado, or it will brown and get mushy.

What's the hardest meal to plan when you're on a ketogenic diet?

If you said lunch, we would agree.Skipping breakfast in favor of a keto bulletproof coffee is common, and you have way more time to cook and eat a scrumptious low carb dinner, but lunch?

Who has time for that during their busy work day?If lunch means heading to one of the best keto fast food places, you're probably bored of eating the same things every week.So it's time you learn the secrets to effortless keto meal prep and get your lunch game on point.

Caveman Chili

This chili is great to make ahead, since it's cooked in the slow cooker for juicy, tender pork. "This is so simple and delicious. I added Parmesan cheese to mine and was able to bring it to work for lunches.

Easy Keto Korean Beef with Cauli Rice

This top-rated keto recipe is ready in 20 minutes, making it perfect for busy weeknight dinners. Cauliflower acts as a great alternative to rice. Simply grate it with a grater or food processor. The ground beef makes it a good source of protein that will keep you feeling full for hours.

Instant Pot Spicy Butternut Squash Soup

This quick and easy butternut squash soup is so flavorful with ginger and brown sugar; and it only takes a few minutes in your Instant Pot," says recipe submitter Fioa. Stick to your diet and indulge in this nutty and creamy soup on a cold winter day. It's a win all around.

Cherry Chicken Lettuce Wraps

Lettuce wraps are a great alternative to all things bread.This asian-inspired wrap is great picnics, or just packing ahead for lunch.

Keto Spaghetti Squash with Bacon and Blue Cheese

Spice up your plain old spaghetti squash with bacon, mushrooms, spinach, and blue cheese.

Low Carb Keto Lasagna

Replacing those carb-heavy lasagna noodles with thinly sliced zucchini not only makes for a healthy, low-carb option, but it also tastes the same when it comes to that soft, cheesy texture. And zucchini is also rich in potassium, anti-inflammatory, easily digestible, low in calories and high in antioxidants and phytonutrients.

Prepare this keto lasagna ahead of time and you'll be a happy camper come lunchtime.

Loaded Cauliflower Bake

This cauliflower casserole is like a loaded baked potato and packs gooey cream cheese, cheddar, bacon, butter and cauliflower. While the secret to this bake is the green onion, you can add your favorite protein and make it different each time.

Easy White Turkey Chili

You may be a keto chili expert, but if you're looking for something a bit different for your hump day lunch, look no further than this classic with a twist. This keto lunch recipe is made with turkey and coconut milk.

Did you know that 93% of coconut milk calories come from fat, including those super healthy saturated fats known as medium-chain triglycerides (MCTs)?

BBQ Pulled Beef Sando

The secret to keto pulled beef is ditching the store-bought BBQ sauce, which is packed with hefty doses of sugar. Pile this baby high on some cloud bread (more on this later!), top with some greens and a dollop of Keto Mayo and you'll be shocked this tasty lunch only clocks in under 5 net carbs.

Portobello Bun Cheeseburgers

There's no need to skip the backyard BBQ to stay in ketosis. This recipe replaces those stale hamburger buns with seasoned portobello mushroom caps for your juicy burger's throne.

Portobello mushrooms contain two types of dietary fiber (beta-glucans and chitin), which each play an important role in helping you manage your weight. With these dietary fibers, your satiety goes up and your appetite does down.

Beberé Enchilada Style Stuffed Peppers

Who says you have to give up enchiladas on keto?Replacing carby tortillas with bell peppers and using beberé, a spice blend of chili peppers, garlic, ginger, basil, cardamom, rue and fenugreek, just to name a few, takes your enchiladas from take out to stand out.

Lemon Herb Low Carb Keto Meatloaf

You can never go wrong with a solid meatloaf it's one of those lunches you drool about at your desk waiting for.But you can go wrong making the same ol' meatloaf too often. So add a bit of variety to your weekly meal prep with this meatloaf made using lemon zest, parsley, oregano and garlic. In one hour you'll have six servings that each come in at just 2 net carbs!

Superfood Meatballs

A superfood enhances the nutritional quality of your diet by providing a wealth of nutrients to reduce your risks of diseases and promote better health. The superfood in these meatballs is chicken liver.

Before you nope out of this recipe, chicken liver boasts tons of health benefits, including:

- Strengthening your immune system
- Promoting better eyesight
- Enhancing fertility
- Fighting stress
- Boosting energy
- Preventing memory loss
- Strengthening teeth and bones

120% of your daily recommended vitamin B12 intake per serving, to help your body make new red blood cells, increase your energy and improve your focus.

Roasted Chicken Stacks

Break out the glass Tupperware because you're going to want to show off these yummy chicken thighs stacked on beds of cabbage and topped with crispy prosciutto to all your coworkers.

Cooking five servings takes less than an hour and reheating them during the week will fill the break room with jealousy.

Curry Chicken Lettuce Wraps

Curry powder is a blend of spices like chili powder, ground coriander, ginger, pepper and the distinctive golden tumeric. These spices are rich in antioxidants and have loads of health benefits including aiding in digestion, cancer prevention and treatment and reducing inflammation.

All you have to do is prepare the chicken the night before, pack the lettuce in your lunch bag separately and assemble during your break for an all-star meal.

It can be difficult to find keto dinner recipes that the whole family will enjoy. Well, the keto dinners below are all delicious and easy to make and even carb addicts will enjoy to eat them!

But most are also easily adjustable by adding rice, potatoes or bread for anyone who doesn't want to eat keto.

Spicy Italian Keto Stuffed Peppers

Bell peppers are one of the best low-carb keto-approved vegetables you can dd to your keto diet plan dinners. While this recipe for Spicy Italian Keto Stuffed Peppers is made with spicy sausage, you could also use sweet (mild) sausage if you prefer. Just be sure to read the label and make sure no extra sugar has been added.

Instead of white rice, which is typical;y called for in stuffed pepper recipes, this recipe uses low-carb riced cauliflower and diced mushrooms, to add filling fiber without loading up on carbohydrates.

Doner Kebab Salad

At its most basic level [the keto diet] is comprised primarily of fat, moderate protein, and low carbohydrates, Eating this way "flips a switch in the body that causes it to preferably burn fat for fuel as opposed to carbohydrates," he explains.

Doner Kebab Salad maximizes on that nutrient profile: Boneless, skinless chicken thighs are coated with a flavorful Greek yogurt sauce that helps the moist cuts of meat retain more flavor. The chicken is served on a bed of cabbage with a heaping serving of Greek yogurt-based tzatziki sauce

Keto Butter Chicken

One of the best things about a low-carb keto diet plan is how versatile it can be. From Italian to Indian, it's possible to eat most cuisines and still meet your carb goals.

Keto Butter Chicken is one incredibly flavorful but simple dinner. Many traditional Indian dishes require hours of simmering and a bounty of ingredients. This dish keeps things weeknight-friendly, while not skimping on the tantalizing warm and spicy notes you love in classic butter chicken.

Zoodles with Avocado Sauce

If you're not familiar with zoodles, they're noodles made with zucchini—the perfect low-carb accompaniment to creamy sauces, tomato sauces, and more. In this Zoodles with Avocado Sauce dish, bright lemon juice combines with fragrant basil and creamy, fat-rich avocado for a luscious sauce. This dish is every bit as good as your favorite fettuccine or spaghett iit just has many fewer carbs.

Chicken Taco Salad

The keto diet works by extremely limiting carbohydrates. This creates a complex metabolic reaction in your body that makes it burn fat instead of glucose a process known as ketosis. "When this biological mechanism is running, and someone is burning more calories than they consume, the body will begin to break down stored body fat for fuel

Fathead Pizza

Eating keto does not mean giving up on pizza; it just means changing how you make it. For this Fathead Pizza, the crust is made with a secret keto-friendly ingredient: almond flour. It's held together with melted mozzarella cheese, cream cheese, and an egg.

Once the crust is all finished, the toppings for a keto pizza can proceed as usual. Look for a sauce that's low in sugar, and sprinkle on your favorite meaty toppings, low-carb veggies like mushrooms and peppers, and a hefty dose of shredded cheese.

Bacon & Egg Sandwich

One of the very best things about the keto diet is that classic breakfast foods like eggs, bacon, ham, and sausage all get the greenlight. Eggs provide a good dose of protein with healthy fats. This "sandwich" recipe calls for a bacon "bun." It's a breakfast-for-dinner keto option that you can pull together in no time.

Sheet Pan Brussels Sprouts with Bacon

If you need to limit protein but crave filling fat, turn to Sheet Pan Brussels Sprouts with Bacon. This dish needs only two ingredients and no more than an hour of your time and it has just the right macro balance with 7 grams of fat, 4 net carbs, and about 8 grams of protein.

Easy Keto Cashew Chicken

Your takeout options might seem limited on the keto plan, but you can recreate some of your dining-out favorites right at home. Keto Connect's Easy Keto Cashew Chicken is a flavor match for your favorite Chinese takeout—but without the carbs from rice, sugary sauce, and breaded coating. Even better, the whole dish is ready in just 15 minutes.

Keto Broccoli Cheese Soup

The primary ingredients broccoli cheese soup are already keto-friendly. But this Keto Broccoli Cheese Soup adds a luscious pour of heavy whipping cream, butter, and xanthan gum a common keto-friendly thickener that can replace high-carb flours.

For busy weeknights, this soup is a satisfying dinner choice. It's ready in under 20 minutes and even the non-keto eaters in the house will love it.

Tenderloin with Horseradish Cream Cheese

Calling all steak lovers: meat eaters tend to love the Keto diet, because it offers plenty of opportunities to have steak and other cuts of red meat. Just add a hefty dose of fats using a flavored mayo or cream cheese, as in this Tenderloin with Horseradish Cream Cheese recipe. To complete this keto dinner, serve it with a side of non-starchy vegetables like asparagus or a spinach salad.

Lemon & Rosemary Chicken

Simple is delicious, and keto can be simple. This Lemon & Rosemary Chicken re uires just seven ingredients but it's so flavorful everyone will think you fussed. Serve with a side of roasted Brussels sprouts (bonus points if you add a mayo dipping sauce), and you've got a low-carb, keto-compliant dinner that everyone at the table will appreciate.

Tenderloin Steak Diane

You can make a keto dinner for two that feels like a restaurant-quality splurge thanks to this recipe for Tenderloin Steak Diane. Whipped cream, butter, and steak sauce form the base of the luscious sauce. Mushrooms (a hardy keto-friendly veggie) turn soft and silky when cooked down in this flavor-packed dish. Serve with roasted broccoli or a side of loaded mashed cauliflower for a full-plate meal.

Baked Keto Chicken Tenders in Buffalo Sauce

Tangy buffalo sauce and creamy blue cheese are a match made in keto heaven. The combination can be used to spice up pork tenderloin, mix with spaghetti squash, or turn typical chicken tenders into an exciting keto dinner.

Buttery Grilled Shrimp

Fish and seafood are rich sources of healthy fat and protein for keto dieters. In this Buttery Grilled Shrimp, double up on the fat content by basting delicate shellfish with butter as they gently cook on the grill. Once they're done, you can eat them as they are or serve with a side of asparagus with melted butter. Save any leftovers to make a simple shrimp salad for the next day's lunch.

It's time to admit something: On a typical diet, soup can get kinda boring (you know, unless you like eating straight-up veggies in broth).The exception to that rule: Keto soup recipes, which are creamy, hearty, and filling (did I say creamy?). The best keto soup recipes contain high-fat.

When you're doing your best to stick to a diet, soup is often a de-facto choice. But more often than not, those soup options are either boring, bland, or from a can. If you've been following the keto diet, and you've done a stellar job of creating meals that are within its high-fat, low-carb stipulations from cooking sheet pan meals to stocking up on snacks to even serving desserts then don't let your soups be any different. On the keto diet, soups can be far from ho-hum.

Instant Pot Zuppa Toscana Soup

It takes all of five minutes to prep this recipe from Krista Rollins at Joyful Healthy Eats and the rest is finished in an Instant Pot. The soup features diced bacon, yellow onion, sausage, cauliflower, and kale in an aromatic broth. "My favorite part about this recipe is the cauliflower.

Crockpot Moroccan Lentil and Chickpea Soup

Not only does this recipe from Half Baked Harvest also require little prep, but it also ensures that you'll get a hearty dish that's still healthy. Tieghan Gerard mixes green lentils, fresh ginger, chickpeas, red bell pepper, and spices together in a crockpot and then waits as the flavors come together over the course of a few hours. "I then topped the soup off with a spoonful of whipped goat cheese, lots of fresh cilantro, mint and lemon juice, plus toasted almonds and pistachios.

Cream of Mushroom Chicken Wild Rice Soup

The key ingredients in this recipe from Half Baked Harvest give it a healthy richness, too, and its other additions of thyme, onion, and garlic are equally irresistible. Gerard also adds boneless, skinless chicken breasts and chicken broth to round out the flavors. "It really doesn't get better than a creamy soup, flavored with mushrooms and loaded with wild rice.

Crockpot Tuscan White Bean and Lemon Soup

Gerard from Half Baked Harvest also makes this colorful recipe for a cozy night in, which features basil pesto, quinoa, sage, kale, white beans, and a parmesan rind. It is especially clear that the parmesan rind is important since it "adds so much flavor without having to add in a million other ingredients." Top it all with even more grated parmesan, and a delicious meal is served.

Mean Green Detox Vegetable Soup

When you need a soup that'll get you back to feeling great or to keep a healthy momentum going this last recipe from Half Baked Harvest is the ticket. It's filled with various vegetables, like broccoli, kale, and carrots, plus herbs and spices for layers of flavors. "I seasoned it up with loads of fresh ginger, garlic, cayenne, soy sauce and a splash of apple cider vinegar," Gerard notes.

Chicken Zoodle Soup

Since the keto diet shies away from pasta, this recipe from Food Faith Fitness can still serve up the flavors of a classic chicken noodle soup but with zucchini instead. It's made with carrots, celery, onion, parsley, and chicken, of course, so you won't even mind the switch. "This homemade chicken broth is keto friendly. "It's just a smattering of delicious herbs, flavors, water and some extra broth for rich flavor.

Broccoli Cheese Soup

Kiser also makes it easy to enjoy the flavors of broccoli and cheese while on a diet thanks to this recipe, which is filled with onion, roasted cashews, and almond milk, too. It all comes together in 15 minutes, which is ideal at any time of the week. "Drain the water from the cashews and place them into a high-powered blender along with the rest of the remaining ingredients.

Instant Pot Keto Chili

Once again, Kiser creates a recipe on Food Faith Fitness that tastes good, comes together easily, and fits in with the keto diet, thanks to this Instant Pot chili. It has celery, onion, lean ground beef, tomatoes, and spices, plus a parsley topping and no beans, even if they might be expected. "All the flavors sitting together in a vat of deliciousness is pretty much just a masterpiece inside your mouth.

Tortilla Soup

It'll be tough not to go for seconds, or even thirds, of this tortilla soup recipe from The Modern Proper, which shreds a rotisserie chicken in red enchilada sauce alongside green chilis, zucchini, corn, onion, garlic, and spices. "It's super satisfying, healthy, quick and inexpensive.

Vegetable Curry Soup

The Modern Proper's vegetable curry soup is yet another colorful and flavorful choice since its ingredients include celery, carrot, ginger, garlic, garam masala, curry powder, coconut milk, and mushrooms.

Everything is added to a large, heavy-bottomed pot to combine, and then the soup is served and topped with cilantro and green onions. "The best part is that dinner is done in 30 minutes and you've got leftovers to be excited about for lunch the next day.

What makes a good dish great? It's all in the sauce, if you ask us. Just think how a tangy dressing can transform a boring salad or how a dry meat dish can be elevated into something mouthwateringly delicious with a spicy marinade or rich gravy. And let's not forget those creamy cheese sauces that, well, just make everything better. Here, 5 keto diet-friendly sauces that will take your dishes to the next level.

Low Carb Thai Peanut Sauce

Low carb, homemade Thai peanut sauce is spicy and delicious on so many different things! It's easy and quick to make - full of healthy fats to keep you satiated until your next meal. Be sure to choose 0 carb ingredients when possible - if not, compare brands to get the ones with the lowest carbs.

Ingredients

- 1/2 cup peanut butter , crunchy
- 3 tablespoons chicken broth ,warm and 0 carb

- 3 tablespoons soy sauce , make sure it's 0 carb per serving
- 3 tablespoons hot sauce , or to taste - I used Louisiana Hot Sauce in this recipe
- 2 tablespoons lime juice
- 1/2 ounce ginger root , grated
- 1/2 tablespoon garlic , minced
- 1/4 teaspoon molasses , unsulfured
- 4 drops pineapple water enhancer , 0 carb
- 1 tablespoon monkfruit , or stevia ...to taste
- 1 tablespoon sesame oil
- 1 teaspoon Fish sauce (nam pla) , optional -as desired

Instructions

1. Whisk all ingredients together until smooth.
2. Place in a non-reactive (glass is best) jar and cover tightly.
3. Let stand at least overnight before using - it helps the flavors to blend.
4. Store in the refrigerator tightly covered.

Notes: Use this spicy Thai peanut sauce on chicken or pork, zoodles, sliced cabbage, or low carb egg noodles.

Pesto Zoodles

Pesto is one of those sauces that enhances pretty much any food it's paired with. Take, for example, zucchini noodles (aka zoodles). A healthy coating of homemade basil pesto takes zoodles to a whole new level. Add some fresh Parmesan and you're golden.

<u>**Ingredients**</u>

Pesto

- 2 cups fresh basil leaves

- 1 garlic clove, smashed

- ⅓ cup pine nuts

- 3 tablespoons grated Parmesan cheese

- ⅓ cup extra-virgin olive oil, or more as needed

- Salt and freshly ground black pepper

Zoodles

- 1 tablespoon extra-virgin olive oil

- 1 sweet onion, thinly sliced

- 4 zucchini, cut into noodles (using a gadget like this)

- Parmesan cheese curls, as needed for garnish

- Red-pepper flakes, as needed for garnish (optional)

Instructions

1. Make the Pesto: In a food processor or blender, pulse the basil, garlic, pine nuts and grated Parmesan until coarsely chopped.

2. With the food processor running, add the olive oil gradually and mix until the pesto is a thick paste. Add more olive oil as needed to adjust the consistency. Add salt and pepper.

3. Make the Zoodles: In a large sauté pan, heat the oil over medium heat. Add the onion and sauté until tender, 4 to 5 minutes. Add the zucchini noodles and sauté until tender, 4 to 5 minutes more.

4. Add the pesto and toss until the noodles are well coated.

5. Serve warm, garnished with Parmesan curls and red-pepper flakes, if using, to taste.

Low Carb BBQ Sauce

This is my most re□uested recipe yet! Enjoy the summer with our low carb BBQ sauce. Less than 2 carbs per serving compared to 18 carbs in store bought! No sugar added, keto friendly.

Ingredients

- 1/4 cup Lakanto Gold brown sugar substitute OR sweetener of your choice (Use code MELISSA20 at checkout to save!)
- 1/4 cup apple cider vinegar
- 1/4 cup white vinegar
- 1/2 cup water
- 2 tablespoons real butter
- 1 can tomato paste
- 1 teaspoon garlic powder
- 1 teaspoon onion powder
- 1 teaspoon dry yellow mustard
- 1 teaspoon salt
- 1 teaspoon cayenne pepper (optional)
- 1 teaspoon liquid smoke (optional)

Instructions

1. In a sauce pan over medium, add sweetener, vinegars and water. Mix until sweetener is dissolved.

2. Add tomato paste and remaining ingredients. Stir until fully combined. Bring to a boil, reduce to simmer.

3. Let simmer about 15 minutes to incorporate all ingredients and build flavor.

NOTES

1. If you like a thinner sauce, add a touch more water until desired thickness is reached.
2. If you like a more sour sauce, add a little more vinegar.
3. Go easy with the li□uid smoke, a little goes a long way!
4. This recipe is very easily adaptable to different sweeteners. Using a white sweetener will result in a sauce that is more red in color.
5. The butter makes a nice glossy finish and helps the sauce adhere to whatever you brush it on.

Creamy Low Carb Alfredo Sauce With Cream Cheese

An easy, creamy Alfredo sauce is made with cream cheese which keeps is low in carbs and gluten-free. This ultimate Parmesan cheese sauce for low carb diets promises delicious authentic Italian taste with every bite.

Ingredients

- 1 cup heavy cream
- 3 oz cream cheese, room temperature
- 2 oz Parmesan cheese, freshly grated
- 2 tbsp butter, room temperature
- 1 large egg yolk
- 1 pinch white pepper
- 1 pinch freshly ground nutmeg
- salt to taste

Additional Flavor Ideas:

lemon zest, parsley, basil, garlic, shallot, white wine, dry sherry, truffle oil, thyme, tarragon

Instructions

1. Gently melt the butter and cream cheese together in a small pot over low heat, whisking to combine.
2. Add 1/4 cup of the heavy cream, turn heat up to medium low, and stir until combined and hot. Add 1/4 of the Parmesan cheese and stir until melted. Alternate adding the heavy cream and Parmesan cheese in the same fashion until all is incorporated.
3. Separate one egg and beat the yolk. When the sauce is hot and bubbling lazily, add the egg yolk while whisking. Turn heat a little lower and continue whisking until the sauce coats the back of a spoon about 1-2 minutes more. Adjust seasonings. Thickens as it cools!
4. Makes about 1 1/2 cups. Serves 4 at approximately 1/3 cup per serving.

Spicy Lemon Herb Sauce

We're all for efficiency in the kitchen. So if we can spend a few minutes making one thing that'll be used throughout the week, we're all for it. Take this spicy lemon herb sauce, which is ready in just 15 minutes. (Amen.) One night, try drizzling it over roasted chicken and veggies to take a standard meal up a notch. Another night, use it as a marinade to flavor fish, pork or tofu. Finally, use it as a dressing to, um, dress up any number of salads, from grains to chicken to greens.

Ingredients

- 1 shallot, peeled and roughly chopped

- 1 garlic clove, peeled and smashed

- 1 bunch parsley, roughly chopped

- 1 bunch mint, roughly chopped

- 1 bunch cilantro, roughly chopped

- 2 lemons, zested and juiced

- ⅓ cup olive oil

- 1 teaspoon salt

- 2 teaspoons freshly ground black pepper

- 1 teaspoon red-pepper flakes, or more to taste

Instuctions

1. In a blender or food processor, pulse the shallot, garlic, herbs and lemon zest to combine.

2. Add the lemon juice and olive oil, then pulse until a smooth sauce forms. Season with salt, pepper and red-pepper flakes.

3. Transfer the sauce to an airtight container and refrigerate until ready to use. The sauce will keep for up to a week.

When you're following a keto or low-carb diet and your sweet tooth cannot be stifled, these sugar-free, low-carb dessert recipes will save the day!

Flourless Avocado Brownies

This recipe by The Castaway Kitchen is perfect for chocolate lovers. These fudgy, low-carb, and dairy-free, avocado brownies are sure to hit the sweet spot without packing on the pounds. The avocado and almond butter pack a ton of healthy fats, which is right in line with the keto diet, and it uses erythitol, the low-calorie sweetener that isn't quite as sweet as sugar. It also uses cacao powder for added richness and flavor.

The best part? These brownies will satisfy your hunger, so you won't want to reach for a second one.

Keto Pistachio Truffles

On Instagram, you see so-called "fat bombs" everywhere, presumably because they're a soft, chewy snack that can satisfy your sweet tooth while still being keto-friendly. They also include such healthy, high-fat ingredients as nut butters, coconut oil, and avocado.

These pistachio keto bombs from I Breathe I'm Hungry are both salty and sweet. They're also ▢uick and easy to make, so you can pop one of these in your mouth and be out the door in about 5 minutes.

Keto Chocolate Chip Muffins

We're not going to encourage you to grab a muffin for breakfast when you can easily whip up one of these healthy on-the-go options instead, but these keto chocolate chip muffins by Fat for Weight Loss are pretty damn delicious regardless. They're only 229 calories and have seven grams of protein. (Pro tip: Use unsweetened dark chocolate to keep the sugar low and the flavor rich.)

Low-Carb Peanut Butter Pie.

A keto-friendly Reese's cup? Sign us up. This low-carb peanut butter pie from Simply So Healthy is perfect for those watching their carb and sugar intake. Using unsweetened cacao powder and stevia, this recipe offers depth and complexity of flavor without being too sweet.

Keto Double Chocolate Chip Cookies

These double chocolate chip cookies from gnom-gnom are intense—they're soft, moist, and totally drool-worthy. You'd never know they were gluten-free and keto-friendly. To help balance out the sweetness, add some sea salt on top for added bite.

Butter Pecan Cookies

Get some keto-friendly fat in with these buttery pecan cookies by All Day I Dream About Food. With only 2.2 grams of net carbs a serving and 22.3 grams of fat, they are great for keto diet macro requirements and they satisfy a sweet craving instantly. Dip them in some tea to make them super soft and yummy.

Keto Chocolates With Macadamia & Sea Salt

Need some V-day inspiration? Whip up these heart-shaped keto chocolates by Ketogasm, which will totally make your partner's heart melt. Plus, they're nice and portion-sized, so you won't feel tempted to overdo it on the sweets and take yourself outside of ketosis. Each serving has just 1 gram of carbs and 13 grams of fat, as well as a mere 120 calories.

Black Walnut Chocolate Chip Keto Low Carb Muffins With Almond Flours

Muffins might seem like breakfast food, but they're also pretty sweet, so they sort of qualify as dessert. And when made with chocolate chips, they definitely do. These muffins by Food Faith Fitness are super soft and decadent, and they only have 5.1 grams of net carbs a serving.

Keto No-Bake Cookies

These no-bake cookies by Sweet As Honey are nice and chocolatey with walnuts to offer a crunchy texture and extra fat to keep you in ketosis. Add in some peanut butter for flavor and to bind, and give them a nice chocolate and coconut cream glaze on top. Each cookie has 4.9 grams of net carbs and 16.9 grams of fat.

Keto Peanut Butter Chocolate Chip Cookies

A match made in heaven? Definitely PB & chocolate. And when inside a soft baked cookie, it's even better. These cookies by Hey Keto Mama are super gooey and rich, and they only cost you 145 calories and 5 grams of net carbs a cookie. Plus there's a nice amount of fat to keep you satisfied with just one.

I'm sure you've already guessed that fat bombs are not actual bombs. Rather, they are wonderful snacks which can provide you with a huge amount of fat.

They have a really high fat percentage and are low in other macros and are of course, keto friendly. They are often made and consumed as a snack and can also be a way to satisfy your sweet tooth once in a while.

They shouldn't of course be a replacement to your regular meals.

On the keto diet, your body uses ketones, gotten from fats as its main energy source. Many times, you might find it a little hard to meet your macronutrient requirements on the keto diet, especially for fat.

Fat bombs are a perfect way to get that extra fat into your diet without falling off ketosis or overeating in general. Here are some reasons to be getting fat bombs in your diet

- They help you meet your macro goals for fat easily
- They can serve as wonderful, sweet tooth satisfying snacks when prepared well
- Fat bombs can help supercharge your brain and body
- They help reduce cravings due to their high fat content
- They can give you a boost into ketosis by adding the extra fat

These are just some of the reasons why fat bombs are a no brainer on keto. But enough of the preaching. Here are 15 delicious keto fat bomb recipes you are going to love.

Keto cheesecake fat bombs

Your regular fat bombs may not taste that good, but the fat bombs on this list are your exception. Starting with this yummy looking keto cheesecake.

Having creamy vanilla for the base layer and thick delicious chocolate for the top section, they look perfect and taste even better. A really awesome way to get more fat into your diet.

Vanilla keto cheesecake fat bombs

This is very similar to the one above, but way less chocolate. You only need 5 simple ingredients to make this recipe, which are cream cheese, coconut oil, butter, vanilla and a nice keto sweetener.

It's super easy to make and gets done pretty quickly. If you want, you can always store some for later. They are a perfect way to satisfy your sweet tooth and also get boosted when it comes to healthy fat intake on keto.

Cookie Dough Fat Bombs

This is another wonderful keto fat bomb recipe worth trying. Made with peanut butter and decorated internally with chocolate chips, this gives a soft, rich and yummy keto fat bomb.

This recipe gives a thick soft chocolate chip-looking cookie that is really easy and fun to snack on

Melt-In-Your-Mouth buttercream Fat Bombs

As the name implies, the joy of this recipe is watching as it melts in your mouth, leaving a cool and rather delicious feeling on your tongue.

This recipe surprisingly only needs 3 ingredients to get the magic going, which are butter, cream cheese and a low carb sweetener. The best part is, it delivers only 0.1g per serving, which is crazy.

You could also enjoy it with some chocolate either by sprinkling some li uid chocolate over it, or dipping it completely. Both seem to go really well.

Chocolate peanut butter fat bombs

Chocolate always seem to make the perfect snack for every situation and this is definitely no exception. This simple chocolate peanut butter fat bomb is made with coconut oil as the base ingredient along with other things that make it amazing.

It is pretty simple and easy to prepare and works as a perfect snack. Just refrigerate for a couple hours after preparation and you're good to go. Since its best served cool, you can always store some for later

Strawberry cheesecake fat bombs

Unlike your regular fat bombs that are mainly just chocolate or vanilla flavoured, this one takes things a bit further by using fruits. Not only are strawberries delicious but also pack a couple of wonderful health benefits.

This simple and easy strawberry cheesecake recipe is creamy, delicious, satisfying and of course freezer friendly so you can always enjoy it la

ter. Definitely a must try.

Dill pickle fat bombs

This keto fat bomb recipe takes thing further by adding some of the best mouth-watering ingredients you could think of. Bacon, cheese and pickles seem like a pretty solid combination to try out.

These delicious bombs can serve as a □uick breakfast, a nice snack or even a side meal. Rich in flavour and high in healthy fats, this will give you the energy and mental boost you need to get you through the day.

Quick and easy cinnamon rolls

Cinnamon is a really wonderful ingredient with very solid health benefits like reduced risk of heart disease. Plus, it's loaded with antioxidants as well. Now, you get to enjoy those health benefits and more in a yummy, healthy snack.

This recipe takes only about 15 minutes to get done and surprisingly delivers only about 0.6g of net carbs per serving. Topped with cream cheese, this fat bomb recipe is kinda hard to resist.

Raspberry cream Heart Jellies

You don't have to wait till valentine before you spread some love or enjoy a recipe like this.

These fat bombs are the perfect blend of delicious and well flavoured. Although they may look like your regular sugar filled snack, these are almost entirely made of fat and are very keto friendly.

Made with sugar-free jello and gelatin powder, they are a perfect go to snack to fill you up with fat and keep you keto boosted for the day.

Cookies and cream (2 ingredient fat bomb)

If you thought 3 ingredients was as low as you could go when it came to fat bombs, then think again. This simple keto recipe is as simple as fat bombs get with only 2 simple ingredients. Yes, 2.

With coconut oil and protein powder, you can make a nice and easy snack loaded with fat. If you want, you could also sprinkle some macadamia nuts over it as a third ingredient.

Either ways, it's a relatively simple and easy fat filled snack to enjoy.

PB & J Fat Bombs

These keto bombs combine the goodness of dried strawberries and raspberries into a fun yummy combination. Made with maple syrup also, it comes out with a nice taste as well as texture.

You only need 10 minutes of prep time to prepare this, refrigerate for a while and you're good to go. This is a wonderful and healthy keto bomb snack to try.

Keto blackberry coconut butter fat bombs

These are like your regular fat bombs, but with blueberries instead. Made with coconut butter, lemon juice and vanilla extract, the combination is set to be a really good and yummy one.

You could prepare this in only 5 minutes and freeze for a few hours until it's ready to go. Its pretty simple and serves as a wonderful snack as well. Overall, you're most definitely going to enjoy this one.

Lemon Cheesecake Keto Fat Bombs

Whenever you're craving something frozen and sweet on the keto diet, this recipe definitely has you covered. Made with lemon juice for zest as well as coconut oil and other ingredients your sweet tooth loves, it's a wonderful snack to enjoy.

You can also top it with blueberries for extra fun. You only need a couple of minutes of prep time and a couple hours to freeze and its ready to be snacked on. It tastes as good as it looks.

Chocolate Peppermint Fat Bombs

These peppermint flavoured keto fat bombs are rather easy to prepare, only needing about 4 minutes of prep time. Covered in chocolate, they make a pretty decent snack.

Generally, they won't be the sweetest thing you'll taste. But if you have somewhat of a sweet tooth, you can always add in some drops of your favourite low carb sweetener to make things better.

Almond Pistachio Fudge

This recipe uses more ingredients than your regular keto fat bomb recipe, but it's definitely worth it. Made by preparing nice almond fudge and topping it with pistachios, this is a wonderful fat filled snack to try out.

When frozen, it gives a nice texture and an even better taste. Plus, you can always still save some for later or share with your friends.

So there you have it. 15 absolutely delicious keto fat bombs to supercharge your body and mind. So whenever you feel like you need a fat filled snack or just want a way to get more fat into your diet, these fat bombs are here for you.

The keto diet focuses mainly on limiting your daily consumption of carbohydrates. Some of the foods that you will have to eliminate from your diet if you intend going keto include, but not limited to the following:

- **Low-fat or diet products:** These are highly processed and often high in carbs.
- **Sugar-free diet foods:** These are often high in sugar alcohols, which can affect ketone levels in some cases. These foods also tend to be highly processed.
- **Grains or starches:** Wheat-based products, rice, pasta, cereal, etc.
- **Fruit:** All fruit, except small portions of berries like strawberries.
- **Beans or legumes:** Peas, kidney beans, lentils, chickpeas, etc.
- **Root vegetables and tubers:** Potatoes, sweet potatoes, carrots, parsnips, etc.
-
- **Unhealthy fats:** Limit your intake of processed vegetable oils, mayonnaise, etc.
- **Alcohol:** Due to their carb content, many alcoholic beverages can throw you out of ketosis.

- **Sugary foods:** Soda, fruit juice, smoothies, cake, ice cream, candy, etc.
- **Some condiments or sauces:** These often contain sugar and unhealthy fat.

You should also try to avoid carb based foods like rice, candy, grains, legumes, sugars, juice, potatoes and even most fruits.

Just in case you find yourself lost or wondering what your daily keto meal plan should look like, then you can take a look at this short and simple guide to help you plan out your meal for the week. They have been compiled to make everything easy for you.

To help get you started, here is a sample ketogenic diet meal plan for one week:

Monday

- **Breakfast:** Bacon, eggs and tomatoes.
- **Lunch:** Chicken salad with olive oil and feta cheese.
- **Dinner:** Salmon with asparagus cooked in butter.

Tuesday

- **Breakfast:** Egg, tomato, basil and goat cheese omelet.
- **Lunch:** Almond milk, peanut butter, cocoa powder and stevia milkshake.
- **Dinner:** Meatballs, cheddar cheese and vegetables.

Wednesday

- **Breakfast:** A ketogenic milkshake.
- **Lunch:** Shrimp salad with olive oil and avocado.

- **Dinner:** Pork chops with Parmesan cheese, broccoli and salad.

Thursday

- **Breakfast:** Omelet with avocado, salsa, peppers, onion and spices.
- **Lunch:** A handful of nuts and celery sticks with guacamole and salsa.
- **Dinner:** Chicken stuffed with pesto and cream cheese, along with vegetables.

Friday

- **Breakfast:** Sugar-free yogurt with peanut butter, cocoa powder and stevia.
- **Lunch:** Beef stir-fry cooked in coconut oil with vegetables.
- **Dinner:** Bun-less burger with bacon, egg and cheese.

Saturday

- **Breakfast:** Ham and cheese omelet with vegetables.
- **Lunch:** Ham and cheese slices with nuts.
- **Dinner:** White fish, egg and spinach cooked in coconut oil.

Sunday

- **Breakfast:** Fried eggs with bacon and mushrooms.
- **Lunch:** Burger with salsa, cheese and guacamole.

- **Dinner:** Steak and eggs with a side salad.

You should make an effort at trying to always switch up on your vegetables and meat consumption from time to time as they are known to provide different health benefits based on what you are consuming.

Now lets recap on the diet.

Must enter the state of ketosis by eliminating carbs from the diet while intaking high fat moderate/low protein.

Must intake fibre of some sort to keep your pipes as clear as ever if you know what I mean.

Once in ketosis protein intake must be at least that of a gram of protein per pound of lean mass.

HOW THE KETOGENIC DIET WORKS IN WEIGHT LOSS

Ketogenic diets force the body to enter into a state called ketosis. The body generally makes use of carbohydrate as its primary source of energy. This owes to the fact that carbohydrates are the easiest for the body to absorb.

However, should the body run out of carbohydrates, it reverts to making use of fats and protein for its energy production. Essentially, the body has a sort of energy hierarchy which it follows.

Firstly, the body is programmed to use carbohydrate as energy fuel when it is available. Secondly, it will revert to using fats as an alternative in the absence of adequate supply of carbohydrate.

Lastly, the body will turn to proteins for its energy provision in when there is an extreme depletion of its carbohydrate and fat stores.

However, breaking down proteins for energy provision leads to a general loss of lean muscle mass.

The ketogenic diet does not fully depend on the calories in, calories out model. This is because the composition of those calories matters due to the hormonal response of the body to different macronutrients.

However, there are two schools of thought in the keto community. While one believes that the amount of calories and fat consumption does not matter, the other contends that calories and fat does matter.

When using a ketogenic diet, you are trying to find a balance point. While calories matter, the composition of those calories also counts. In a ketogenic diet, the most important factor of the composition of those calories is the balance of fat, protein and carbohydrates and how each affects insulin levels.

This balance is very important because any rise in insulin will stop lipolysis. Therefore, you need to eat foods that will create the smallest rise in insulin. This will help to keep your body in the state of burning stored body fat for fuel - lipolysis.

The body can normally go into a ketosis state by itself. This is often the case when you are in a fasting state such as when you are sleeping. In this state, the body tends to burn fats for energy while the body carries out it repairs and growth while you sleep.

Carbohydrates generally make up most of the calories in a regular meal. Also, the body is inclined to make use of the carbohydrate as energy as it is more easily absorbable. The proteins and fats in the diet are thus more likely to be stored.

However, in a ketogenic diet, most of the calories come from fats rather than carbohydrates. Since ketogenic diets have low amount of carbohydrates, they are immediately used up. The low carbohydrate level causes an apparent shortage of energy fuel for the body.

As a result of this seeming shortage, the body resorts to its stored fat content. It makes a shift from a carbohydrate-consumer to a fat-burner. The body however does not make use of the fats in the recently ingested meal but rather stores them up for the next round of ketosis.

As the body gets more familiar to burning fat for energy, fats in an ingested meal become used up with little left for storage.

This is why the ketogenic diet uses a high amount of fat consumption so that the body can have enough for energy production and also still be able to store some fat. The body needs to be able to store some fat otherwise it will start breaking down its protein stores in muscles during the ketosis period.

In fasting periods - such as during ketosis, in between meals and during sleep - the body still needs a constant supply of energy. You have these periods in your normal day and therefore you need to consume enough amounts of fat for your body to use as energy.

If there are no ade☐uate amounts of stored fat, the proteins contained in your muscle become the next option for the body to use as energy. It is therefore important to eat enough to avoid this scenario from taking place.

The main goal of a ketogenic diet is to mimic the state of starvation in the body. Ketogenic diets deprive the body of its preferred immediate and easily convertible carbohydrates by restricting and severely cutting back on carbohydrate intake. This situation forces it into a fat burning mode for energy production.

FOODS YOU CAN EAT ON A KETOGENIC DIET FOR WEIGHT LOSS

While on a ketogenic diet, it is very important to ensure that one eat within the restrictions of the diet. This is vital so as for the individual to be able to remain in a state of ketosis.

Going out of ketosis can be as simple as eating one or two meals that are not recommended on the diet. However, coming back into ketosis is another different story entirely. This can often takes days or weeks depending on how strict you become when you get back on the diet.

Meals in a ketogenic diet comprise of three basic food types. These are the:

- fruit or vegetable
- protein-rich food
- fat source

Fats

Ketogenic diets by nature involve the consumption of increased amounts of fats in the diet. They can come in as part of the cooking process or as sauces and dressings.

The best types of fats are those medium-chain triglycerides (MCTs). These include both MCT oil and coconut oil. Medium-chain triglycerides are easily metabolized to produce ketones. Some other equally good fats for ketosis include:

- Omega-3 and Omega-6 fatty acids
- Salmon, Shellfish, Trout, Tuna
- Monounsaturated and Saturated fats
- Olive oil, Avocado, Butter, Cheese, Red palm oil, Egg yolks
- Non-hydrogenated oils (when cooking)
- Coconut oil, Beef tallow, Non-hydrogenated lards
- High oleic
- Safflower oils, Sunflower oils
- Other fat sources:
- Chicken skin, Coconut butter, Peanut butter, Fat on meats

Proteins

When buying your protein foods, always try to choose grass-fed, organic and humanely raised meat and wild-caught seafood. Apart from offering more nutrients, they have not been exposed to added hormones, antibiotics, and other potential toxins.

Meat

The ketogenic diet accepts basically any type of meat. There is no discrimination about the type of cut or preparation.

Beef, Goat, Lamb, Pork, Veal, Venison

Poultry

Any type of poultry is also allowed by the diet. You can improve the content of the meal by leaving the skin on. However, breading and batter should not be used in the preparation of poultry as they are usually high in carbohydrates. Other than that, you can prepare your poultry to your liking.

Chicken, Duck, Game hen, Goose, Ostrich, Partridge, Pheasant, Quail, Squab, Turkey

Seafood

Another great source of protein is seafood. Seafood is a great source of omega-3 fatty acids. They also have high amounts of minerals and vitamins to help keep you well-nourished and healthy.

Clams, Crab, Lobster, Mussels, Oysters, Prawns, Scallops, Shrimp, Snails

Fish

Fish have good amounts of omega-3 fatty acids. You should go for fish that are caught in the wild and also in mercury-free areas.

Ahi, Catfish, Cod, Flounder, Halibut, Herring, Lobster, Mackerel, Mahi mahi, Mussel, Salmon, Sardines, Scallops, Snapper, Squid, Swordfish, Trout, Tuna, Walleye.

Vegetables

Vegetables are the primary source of carbohydrate on a ketogenic diet. When you are buying vegetables always opt for the organically grown vegetables. Also, the dark leafy vegetables contain the least amount of carbohydrates with good nutritional value.

Arugula, Asparagus, Bok choy, Broccoli, Cabbage, Cauliflower, Celery,Collard greens, Endive, Garlic, Kale, Kelp, Lettuce, Mushrooms, Onions, Peppers, Radishes, Seaweed, Spinach, Swiss chard, Watercress

Milk and Dairy Products

These are very essential in a ketogenic diet. Grass-fed and organic source are more preferable. The full fat variety is better suited for the ketogenic diet than the fat-free and low-fat verities.

Butter, Cheddar, Crème fraîche, Heavy cream, Mozzarella, Sour cream, Cream cheese, Mascarpone cheese, Cheeses, Hard cheeses

Nuts

Moderate amounts of nuts and seed are allowed on the ketogenic diet. Nuts and seed are rich in protein, fats, and carbohydrates. The total fat, protein and carbohydrate content of the nut varieties should be checked and added to the total daily calorie calculation.

Roasted nuts and seeds are the best. Anything that may cause harm or interfere with ketosis in the body has been removed from them through the roasting process.

Nuts should be used mostly as a snack

Almonds, Macadamia, and Walnuts are some of the best

Some nuts have high content of omega-6 fatty acid which can cause inflammation in the body

However, they can hold some people back from their goals. If your weight loss is purely your purpose of using the ketogenic diet, then it would be advisable to remove nuts and seeds to improve your results.

Almonds, Brazil nuts, Hazelnuts, Pine nuts, Macadamia nuts, Pecans, Pili nuts, Pumpkin seeds, Sesame seeds, Sunflower seeds, Walnuts

<u>Herbs and Spices</u>

After some time on the ketogenic diet, the foods may start to become boring. Adding spices to your meals can however help to spice things up. You can add fresh and dry spices to your meals and even beverages so that they become more enticing and exciting to the palate.

Spices and fresh herbs are some of the most nutrient-dense foods on the planet you can eat. Adding spices to your meal doesn't only add more flavors to the meals but also offer a lot of various health benefits to your body.

Spices contain carbohydrates thus you should ensure to add them to your daily carbohydrate count. Also, endeavor to check the labels of pre-made spice mixes for their accurate carbohydrate content as they usually contain added sugars.

Salt also enhances flavors. It is best you chose high quality sea salt instead of traditional table salt. Unprocessed salts such as Celtic or Himalayan sea salt provide you with more than eight trace minerals that your body need to perform optimally.

Anise, Annatto, Basil, Bay leaf, Black pepper, Caraway Cardamom, Cayenne pepper, Celery seed, Chervil, Chili pepper, Chives, Cilantro, Cinnamon, Cloves, Coriander, Cumin, Curry, Dill, Fenugreek, Galangal, Garlic, Ginger, Lemongrass, Licorice, Mace, Marjoram, Mint, Mustard seeds, Oregano, Paprika, Parsley, Peppermint, Rosemary, Saffron, Sage, Spearmint, Star anise, Tarragon, Thyme, Turmeric, Vanilla beans

Sweeteners

Adding artificial sweeteners to your meals can help in curbing cravings for carbohydrates and sweets. Sweeteners help a lot of people to be able to adhere to the ketogenic diet.

However, natural sweeteners such as honey, maple syrup, and agave raise blood sugar levels which does not only cause inflammation but can also kick you out of ketosis.

Always go for the liquid form of sweeteners as they do not have binders like dextrose and maltodextrin. Dextrose is an anti-caking agent and is a form of sugar. Maltodextrin on the other hand is a bulking agent which has higher glycemic index (110) than table sugar (52).

The following is a list of recommended sweeteners which have little effect on blood sugar.

Allulose, Blended sweeteners (Swerve, Lakanto, Sukrin), Erythritol, Monk fruit, Stevia, Stevia glycerite (a thick liquid form of stevia), Sucralose, Xylitol

Beverages

Using a low carbohydrate diet like the ketogenic diet has a diuretic effect on the body. Carbohydrates draw water to them which cause water retention in the body. However, the reduced carbohydrate intake in a ketogenic diet leads to a lot water loss as less water is retained in the body and more is excreted.

This diuretic effect can easily lead to dehydration. Therefore you need to drink a lot of water - well above the recommended intake of 8 glasses - when you are on a ketogenic diet. This will help you to reduce the risk of bladder pain and urinary tract infections.

Besides water, you can add other types of beverages like coffee and teas to help keep your hydrated throughout the day. Both of these do not significantly affect the ketosis state.

However, the added substances like sugar and milk might affect the ketosis state. As a result, it would be best to avoid the sugar completely and use either full cream or artificial sweeteners together with your coffee or tea.

Another way to increase your beverage intake is to make vegetable juice by combining varieties of the approved vegetable types. You can also use a power smoothies or protein shakes instead of a fruit smoothies as the fruits contain sugars (fructose) that can kick you out of ketosis.

Below are some additional beverages you can consume to help keep you hydrated:

Unsweetened almond milk, Unsweetened cashew milk, Unsweetened coconut milk, Unsweetened hemp milk, Green tea, Herbal tea, Organic caffè Americano (espresso with water), Mineral water.

That is pretty much it! It takes dedication to no eat carbs through out the week as a lot of foods have carbs, but remember you will be rewarded greatly for your dedication. You must not stay in the state of ketosis weeks on end as it is dangerous and will end up with your body turning to use protein as a fuel source which is a no no. Hope it's helped and good luck dieting!

It's difficult, if you are just starting out looking for a diet that works for you, to know where the truth lies in this debate; if the scientists can't sort it out then how are you going to?

The plain truth is that you'll need to educate yourself, weigh up the arguments, then follow your own best judgement.

My experience has been largely positive but you will, no doubt, have heard of friends having problems on low carbohydrate diets for one reason or another.

There is no such thing as a miracle diet and most of them are just variations on a theme but all ketogenic-type diets are based upon a very specific principle and that principle has been demonstrated to induce weight loss in many people. Perhaps you should try to base your opinion on the available evidence and not on anecdotes. It's your body and your health, after all.